Community-Based
Medical Education

Community-Based Medical Education
Towards a shared agenda for learning

Noel Boaden
Emeritus Professor of Continuing Education and
Senior Research Fellow, University of Liverpool, UK

John Bligh MD FRCGP
Professor of Medical Education, University of Liverpool, UK

with a foreword by

Sir Kenneth Calman
Formerly Chief Medical Officer

A member of the Hodder Headline Group
LONDON • SYDNEY • AUCKLAND
Co-published in the USA by
Oxford University Press Inc., New York

First published in Great Britain in 1999 by
Arnold, a member of the Hodder Headline Group,
338 Euston Road, London NW1 3BH

http://www.arnoldpublishers.com

Co-published in the United States of America by
Oxford University Press Inc.,
198 Madison Avenue, New York, NY10016
Oxford is a registered trademark of Oxford University Press

British Library Cataloguing in Publication Data
A catalogue record for this book is available from the British Library

Library of Congress Cataloging-in-Publication Data
A catalog record for this book is available from the Library of Congress

ISBN 0 340 70012 2

1 2 3 4 5 6 7 8 9 10

Commissioning Editor: Fiona Goodgame
Production Editor: James Rabson
Production Controller: Priya Gohil
Cover Design: Terry Griffiths

Typeset in 10/12 pt Minion by Phoenix Photosetting, Chatham, Kent
Printed and bound in Great Britain by J.W. Arrowsmith Ltd, Bristol

What do you think about this book? Or any other Arnold title?
Please send your comments to feedback.arnold@hodder.co.uk

Contents

Foreword

How health care is to be provided is one of the most widely discussed topics by the public, professionals, patients and politicians. Its shape, structure, mode of access and quality are all relevant to the care of patients. Over the past few years the emphasis has changed and health care is now seen to be more community-based and patient-focused. It is within this context that the delivery of medical education, indeed all professional education, should be considered. Medical education itself is in the process of significant change at all levels. The Undergraduate Course, the early Postgraduate Training, Specialist Training and continuing professional development, have all seen important changes which are relevant to the context in which medicine is practised.

The purpose of medical education is to provide a group of well-trained doctors who can provide both individual and population care to patients and the community. It therefore has a clear focus, and this must be seen both in the context of health, and of illness. There needs to be a greater focus on the former, as well as the traditional emphasis on the latter. In addition to this, as more health care is delivered in a community context, so education has to be set in the same way, and those in training need to think about the community as part of the learning environment.

With the purpose clearly defined, and some of the settings clear, it is evident that the process of medical education is also undergoing a process of change. Methods of education, the development of the curriculum, the content of the process and methods of assessment are all being reconsidered. The emphasis is on learning, and the teacher in this sense is seen as someone who facilitates that process. There is greater emphasis on project work, self-assessment, and a consideration of the specific needs of individual learners.

With this in mind the setting of the learning process is also changing. Traditionally this has been in hospitals, and particularly in acute care settings. Yet a great deal of the work of many doctors will be in the community, and dealing with long-term illness. Doctors need to consider issues in a population sense, and in the environment in which the patient lives and works. For that reason the shift to community education has to be welcomed, together with a much greater emphasis now on multi-disciplinary teaching. Working in teams and problem-solving are very much part of the learning process. This needs to be set in the context of improving the quality of patient care, the real outcome of the educational process.

The process just outlined is the substance of this book. It considers community-based and team-based learning and shows how these two processes can bring benefits to the educational process, and thus to patient care. It links the setting of health care delivery, predominantly in the community, to the educational process. It is a book therefore that challenges existing assumptions, and provides very good examples for all those concerned with the education of professional staff in the NHS to consider in detail.

Sir Kenneth Calman
Formerly Chief Medical Officer

Introduction

The relationship between the delivery of health care services and the education of the staff who will provide those services is a complex one in all countries, whether their systems are well developed or still developing. In the developed world, health care services have a widely established capacity to deliver very high quality care utilising the most advanced medical techniques and practices. Such development has required the creation of large-scale hospitals and the employment of highly trained medical specialists with large teams of supporting staff to facilitate their work. At the same time such systems continue to deliver a large array of other health services, usually within the community, employing generalist doctors supported by diverse teams of staff. The two sectors of health care have a close, but complex relationship, but the more technical medicine and serious acute care tends to enjoy both the larger share of the resources being used, and higher status among health care professionals. One result is that professional education has been relatively dominated by the demands of the acute hospital sector.

In contrast, the developing countries have health care systems which reflect a much earlier phase in the evolution of health care. The highly technical services form a much smaller proportion of their overall care systems, and are limited to the few major urban centres which can support highly specialised care in countries with relatively dispersed rural populations. The community-based, generalist services consequently have a more significant role in that they are usually the only source of health care for large numbers of people. This is reflected in the availability of professional staff. There are of course highly trained doctors, many trained in the medical schools of developed countries or by doctors from such countries, and staffing the centres of acute care. By contrast, the extensive community services have few generalist family practitioners and are more dependent on nurses or other less highly trained groups of staff, or in many cases on lay workers. Pressures on medical education are divided between the development of highly qualified specialists and the needs of extensive community-based care.

The expectation until very recently was that the developing countries would evolve along the established path of development experienced in the developed countries. Sophisticated health care provision would accompany urbanisation and industrialisation, and professional medical education would expand to meet the need for highly trained doctors. Community-based care would also develop, but as in developed countries would not enjoy parity of status in professional terms. This expected pattern of development has been increasingly questioned over recent years as economic development has failed to deliver the capacity to afford such health care and done little to limit health care needs. Ironically, the same factors have also been felt in the more developed countries where the demand for health care, and the cost of sophisticated treatment, have become too high, certainly for many politicians. The result is that both kinds of system are concerned to formulate and implement health care reform. At the same time governments and the professions are seeking changes in professional education for health care workers which better fit the emerging and future staffing needs.

Clearly this is a complex process. Some would argue that the relationship between the two elements is driven by changes in health care which prompt consequential changes in professional education (Field and Kinmonth 1995) with some commentators adopting that causal argument in support of the case for educational reform (Hennessy and Tomlinson 1994). Others appear to consider that developments in the education of health care professionals will stimulate changes in the provision of health care, although the argument that a 'health system as massive as ours cannot be changed without changing how physicians are educated at all levels' (Todd 1992, p. 1133) acknowledges the connection but implies no particular direction in the causal relationship.

In any case the debate is somewhat academic. Both views seem somewhat optimistic when set against the history of development in systems of health care and health care education which provides more evidence that the two are as often incongruent as they are effectively aligned. Changes in health care systems in the past, like so many areas of public policy, have been irregular in frequency and modestly incremental in scale. Wider structural change of necessity does not occur often and while innovations in health care practice are more frequent, they often take many years to diffuse through the system to become widely used by the professionals involved (Stocking 1985). This pattern has itself shown signs of changing in recent years in some developed countries under the pressures of economic constraint and political conservatism. Structural change has become more frequent, outstandingly in the case of the British National Health Service, while modern technology is assisting the more rapid diffusion of innovatory practice, with both changes making health care systems generally more volatile.

The evidence on medical education contrasts sharply with this pattern, showing a much more conservative history and considerable resistance to change even in the more recent volatile health care climate. This is well illustrated by the General Medical Council of the United Kingdom in reviewing the history of medical education and finding the same reforming themes occurring over a period of more than a hundred years without significant changes being made (General Medical Council 1993). Their review is echoed in commentary from the United States where studies of recommendations for reform and their impact on health care education confirm the innate conservatism of the system of professional education (Enarsun and Burg 1992).

There is no need to take sides in a debate about causation. Whichever view is taken, the important fact is that health care education and health care are closely related, and should ideally operate together. The historical evidence suggests that they were perhaps more congruent in an earlier period when the medical profession asserted considerable influence over both (Grumbach 1995). Certainly, medical education developed to meet the clinical needs of the acute, hospital sector of the health care system. At the same time that emphasis served the interests of the profession, providing strong legitimation for the claim to professional status. More recently, professional influence has weakened in relation to health care, though not in relation to education, removing one factor which had traditionally helped maintain congruity.

This weakening of professional influence in health care has arisen because many developed countries are being moved towards radical reform of their health care systems by pressures of cost and the political implications of meeting such cost whether from tax revenue or through medical insurance. In face of such pressures, professional influence, particularly if perceived as being used to inhibit change, becomes less acceptable. New reform processes are taking place which by-pass some of the professional consultation which would once have occurred with the result that reform often goes ahead, and takes forms which do not always command professional approval or support. One implication tends to be a greater demand for professionals to adjust their organisation, their clinical practice and their care delivery to meet externally imposed changes than was traditionally the case. Another consequence is a clear challenge to the professions to exercise their control over medical education to prepare doctors for the new health care models being introduced. In such circumstances it is hard to disagree with Todd when he says that 'nothing is more important to the future health of our nation or the success of our profession than a medical educational system that is relevant, responsive and responsible' (1992, p. 1134). Failure to deliver such education could lead to more externally imposed change in professional education, a change which could ultimately undermine formal claims to professional status.

The challenge is made more difficult by the fact that professional education often reflects the needs of a past situation, serving the professional claims and values which were the basis of an earlier system and which sustained the original claims to professional legitimacy. Public acceptance of professional control of health care education was understandable in a naturally stable health care system, or one in which the professions could use their wider influence to secure stability and congruity between care and education. For a long time, however, medical education has been known not to serve all aspects of health care equally well. It failed to track the incremental changes in patterns of illness and consequent health care and could not supply the skill mix essential to new patterns of care delivery. The more volatile situation of recent years has exacerbated that situation, and professional educators and practitioners are having to cope with economic, social and political factors assuming more significance in health care decisions. This becomes more marked when reform is changing the emphasis of health care, between sectors and between geographical areas, changes which challenge directly the traditional, and prevailing, patterns of professional dominance. These pressures are further compounded by the fact that both the context and character of health care seem likely to continue to change significantly into the foreseeable future.

The gap between medical education and the health care system is evident in a number of ways. In the United States there is clearly a deep concern at the inadequate numbers of doctors leaving medical schools equipped and motivated to take up careers in family medicine despite the widely recognised need for more family doctors within the system (Campos-Outcalt *et al.* 1995). Ironically, that continuing demand for more family doctors reflects a situation in primary care which has been understood for some time but not been met. Now that it is being met, the kind of doctors needed are already changing amid concerns about the nature of medical practice in the twenty-first century and the clinical and other skills that will become relevant as changes continue (Greenlick 1995). In Britain the debate addresses different issues. Here primary care has occupied a central role with large numbers of medical graduates going into general practice and since the improvements in general practice of the mid-1960s recruitment to family medicine has not been a problem. The problem here arises more from the fact that satisfactory recruitment occurs despite wide recognition that conventional existing medical education has not provided a good preparation for general practice. The result has been a need to develop extended postgraduate training to learn the new skills and approaches more appropriate to community-based practice and 'unlearn' some of the lessons from medical school. This postgraduate system has adequately served 20 years of relatively stable practice, but the extensive changes in primary care and the wider NHS introduced in the 1990s are creating a situation in which recruitment of new family doctors is declining, with evidence that many existing doctors are not adapting well to the new demands being placed upon them. As in the United States, adjusting to current needs is being overtaken by an emerging discussion about the nature and needs of community-based general practice into the next century (Irvine 1993).

These varied pressures are leading everywhere to efforts being made to bring professional education into closer congruence with the health care system which provides its ultimate rationale and legitimacy. These efforts are difficult because the two systems to be reconciled work under quite different constraints and sources of influence in their development. Health care is essentially a political matter, given the volume of resources involved in its supply, and the distributive and redistributive implications of its funding, organisation and practice. The form of politics varies, being dominated by conventional politics in those systems where health care is funded largely from tax revenues, and by the decisions of insurance companies in systems where private insurance forms a significant basis for access to care. In some cases public and private systems coexist, catering for different clienteles within a single country, making the politics even more complicated. Whatever the system of funding, the imperatives of escalating need and demand for health care in all countries have to be reconciled with the economic and political limitations on what is affordable, making health care rationing inevitable, and continuing reform of the health care system highly probable.

In contrast, in most countries the medical profession has been accorded a large degree of independent control over medical education, distancing the process from public politics and from more direct government intervention. The result is an education system dominated by professional politics and consequently reflecting the structures of power and influence which prevail within the profession. Such structures often reflect patterns of professional dominance established in the past, and those who have been influential have successfully retained their influence despite changes in professional practice and the other demands generated by systemic changes within health care. There was a time when those same influential professionals would have asserted their influence to inhibit such external changes in health care, but the recent reduction in that external influence has allowed the two systems to move further apart.

The current need is to restore, or establish, greater congruence between the two systems. Inevitably, given the nature of the two systems, and the imperatives operating to change health care, this will involve changes in medical education. It is becoming apparent that changes will be imposed if the profession fails to make the changes deemed necessary. Such changes must, inevitably, pose a serious challenge to the long-established patterns of professional influence within medical education. The level of change involved may be more radical for two reasons. One is the lack of change over such a long period, suggesting a need for more substantial change to catch up with intervening developments. The other, which may involve even wider changes, is that the current resource-driven debate within health care is forcing consideration of more radical changes to both health care and medical education, many such changes posing a direct challenge to the traditional intra- and inter-professional hierarchy and patterns of practice.

OUTLINE OF THE TEXT

The remainder of the text addresses these broad questions and considers the changes needed in medical education if it is to be more effective in preparing tomorrow's doctors to meet the challenges and exploit the opportunities provided by community-based practice. The first three chapters provide a more detailed examination of the arguments sketched earlier in this introduction. Chapter 1 deals with the health care delivery systems for which medical education has to prepare doctors. It discusses the constraints under which health care systems in developed countries are labouring and the constant emphasis being placed on community-based care in order to manage those constraints. Chapter 2 moves to the other side of the equation to look at medical education. A brief review of the history is followed by an examination of some recent efforts to reform medical education, concluding that the limited changes made have failed to keep pace with those occurring within health care systems, leaving a widening gap between the two systems. Chapter 3 moves from general reform to consider some of the specific efforts made within medical education to meet the need for a more community-based curriculum. Examples from the developing world are used to illustrate a different perspective, while others drawn from a number of developed countries are used to illustrate the limits of existing reforms. There is an apparent confusion between new teaching methods and a major change in the orientation and purpose of medical education which points up the need for a more radical debate about reform.

Chapters 4 to 6 examine the basic elements which should underlie that debate. Chapter 4 considers the many aims and objectives which might be served by the development of community-based education, ranging from improvements in conventional medical recruitment and practice to the development of much more radical practice within the community. This is a difficult area of debate as it impacts much more closely on established professional interests than do other issues of method and process. They are also important, however, and the next two chapters consider two central issues which need to be consistent with agreement about aim and purpose. Chapter 5 considers where medical education should occur and examines the wide range of community-based settings which might address the varied aims and objectives considered. Chapter 6 in turn considers the teaching and learning methods and approaches which will need to be developed in order to achieve agreed new aims and objectives, and sensibly exploit the opportunities provided by the new settings.

Chapters 7 to 9 move forward from this discussion to consider three specific concerns which are highly relevant if curriculum reform is to meet the demands which future community-based health care systems will place on doctors. Chapter 7 recognises the multi-professional character of such health systems and examines the consequent need for inter-professional education in professional development. The practicalities involved in implementing such changes are also considered. Chapter 8 moves the discussion further in arguing the importance for professionals of understanding the context within which inter-professional work is undertaken. Future doctors and other health care professionals will need a much more developed understanding of, and capacity to deal with, both intra- and inter-agency models of practice which are needed in community-based care. Chapter 9 moves the discussion from a concentration on initial professional education to consider the importance of continuing professional development. This is important in the development of community-based practice but is also vital to the continued adaptation of that practice as health care systems continue to respond to changing public needs and to the constraints within which they continue to operate.

Finally, Chapter 10 suggests that the future might be considered in a much more radical way and that community-based education can serve that more radical agenda, and may need to do so. It is argued that only when the discussion moves beyond incremental changes and breaks free of the constraints of past practice will the really radical opportunities be grasped.

1

Changing health care systems

PRESSURES FOR CHANGE

The principal focus of the work which follows is medical education in its broadest sense, but it is clear from the Introduction that such a focus must be wide enough to encompass the changes in health care which are promoting educational reform. This is particularly important when those changes are as widespread, and as radical, as they have been in recent years in several countries. The pressures for such change arise from the difficulty all countries are experiencing in meeting the seemingly endless growth in the need and demand for health care with the limited resources which governments, and people, are willing to spend on health care. This pressure is very obvious in publicly provided systems such as the National Health Service in Britain, where universal free access to care and the tax burden involved in paying for care make health a central focus of political debate. It is equally apparent in the United States where reform of the public system of care has been under debate and where the quite different insurance-based system of funding is driving decisions about priorities and about the organisation of health care (Grumbach 1995).

Whatever their system for funding health care, all countries with developed health care systems are facing similar pressures arising from a number of sources. One source is the continuing development of the capacity of medicine to prevent, treat and cure an ever-widening range of conditions. Another is the fact that public expectations about their health care have risen steadily with the development of medicine and the provision of organised health care, encouraging people to expect that new medical treatments will be universally available. This mixture of increased capability and rising expectations is exacerbated by other pressures. Among the most significant of these pressures are the changes in the population structure affecting most developed countries, caused partly by medical advances, but also by more general improvements in social and economic conditions. All these countries have successfully dealt with the traditional epidemic diseases of earlier less-developed periods through a combination of public health measures and immunisation programmes. They have also developed a high capacity for handling many of the most life-threatening episodes of acute illness which continue to occur. Taken together, these developments have greatly extended life expectancies for many people, leading to a consequent growth in overall population numbers. Life expectancy in most developed countries has extended over the last fifty years so that most people now live into their late sixties and many will survive into their eighties in sharp contrast to the situation as little as 25 years ago.

Such ageing populations have a number of consequences. One is the economic pressure on individuals to maintain their economic position through long periods of retirement, and the enormous pressure on state retirement schemes, both of which have consequences for the quality of life and health experienced in later years. Another is the demands imposed on informal carers of the elderly and chronically sick by the extended periods of care now involved, carers who are, by definition, themselves getting older and less able to provide the support which they once might have done. Another stems from the increased demand for health care expressed by older people stemming from the patterns of morbidity which are known to increase with age (Rowlands *et al.* 1997). Most of these demands were disguised in the past by earlier mortality. This situation encouraged, or at least allowed, the health care system to develop in ways which focused on acute care and which paid significantly less attention to treating the chronic conditions associated with older patients. The implications of this changing demography for the health care system are thus considerable in terms of the kinds of service now required, the growing scale of demand for such services and the need for significant changes in established patterns of health care if they are to be met. Many of the conditions which inhibit or undermine the quality of life of older people are not the acute conditions which involve the leading edge of medical advance and the dominant interests within the profession. They are the chronic conditions which, if experienced over a longer lifespan, can have much more drastic consequences than they had in the past, imposing greater strain on less developed support services. The wider and more equitable provision of well-understood, basic, but often not well-established, services is what is required, often widening the definition of health care to include related areas of social and community care.

The redistribution involved in this change of emphasis is not easy to achieve in any circumstances. It is made even more difficult by the fact that direct demands for acute health care continue to arise from other features of modern life in developed countries. The traditional diseases may have been overcome but in their place have emerged a wide range of new diseases, many associated with the lifestyles of the late twentieth century. Heart disease and cancer are among the diseases which now contribute disproportionately to death rates, but also have dramatic impact on the quality of life, and patterns of morbidity, creating significant consequent demands for health care. Other diseases arise from the increased scale of city dwelling, and the dominance of motor transport giving rise to environmental pollution on an extensive scale. These prevailing pressures are also leading to a higher incidence of psychiatric illnesses of various kinds, which are exacerbated in their effect by changes in public attitudes about appropriate ways to treat such conditions. These are pushing the health care system to shift treatment for such conditions out of the hospital sector into the community, relying on a mixture of informal and professional care to maintain those who suffer mental illness. These very obvious pressures are compounded by the fact that in some areas some traditional diseases are re-emerging as a result of modern social and economic inequalities and the impact of some urban lifestyles.

These pressures on the demand side of health care confront a system designed to meet an earlier style of demand which involved well-established patterns of treatment and care, managed and organised to reflect the dominant influences within medicine. All the developed health care systems provide a broad spectrum of care, but within that spectrum distinct priorities have emerged and been encouraged over the years, with the allocation of resources heavily skewed in favour of some forms of care rather than others. These patterns reveal the traditional emphasis on acute hospital care and the relatively limited resourcing of care in the community designed to deal with chronic and continuing care needs. In a period where the context of health care has become more volatile, and the demands on the system have changed, the established pattern of care delivery can be an obstacle to the delivery of effective care and can certainly inhibit changes in the pattern of care. In a system where the criteria for judging health care are being extended to include efficiency as well as effectiveness, managing new services within old structures can certainly get in the way of delivering care more cost-effectively. Given the labour-intensive character of all forms of health care, all of these pressures are concentrated in difficult decisions on the staffing of health care and in handling the organisational and professional consequences of change.

Large numbers of staff are employed in the delivery of modern health care, ranging from the highly trained professional doctors to the ancillary staff essential to the functioning of large hospitals. In between are a range of other 'semi-professional' staff such as nurses, physiotherapists and managers, all playing inter-dependent, key roles in the delivery of complex health care. Several features of such large-scale and complex systems are important in the context of reform. One is the difficulty of creating the appropriate formal structures within which this range of staff can be effectively organised. The scale of health care provision and its labour-intensive character demand a degree of formality and hierarchy in organisation to provide the control and supervision essential to the non-professional staff. At the same time professional staff demand, and in some cases require, substantial autonomy from such formality and hierarchy in their practice. The 'semi-professionals' who fall in between are often seeking professional status and the autonomy which that brings, but meanwhile continue to require supervision, although many operate in situations in the community where supervision is difficult. The varied conditions of work inherent in these differences are often associated with different motivations for working and changing aspirations in terms of the contribution to changing health care that each group feels it might make. The challenges to the financial and human resource managers responsible for delivering effective, affordable and equitable health care are enormous.

Meeting these challenges is made more difficult by the inter- and intra-professional relationships which have become established within health care as it has developed. One feature of those relationships is the dominant role of the medical profession within the overall system, a dominance which has traditionally extended outside their legitimate professional concern with clinical issues into influence over the organisation, management and prioritising of care (Klein 1989). The most obvious effect of this dominance is the gap between doctors and other workers within health care in terms of their status and influence. This has led to the containment of non-medical professions into limited roles, traditionally regarded as ancillary to medicine, rather than them being accepted as independent professions in their own right capable of making a much wider contribution to health care. That overall medical dominance does not mean that there are no divisions within medicine. Influence patterns within the profession are reflected in a clear hierarchy of medical specialties which has emerged over the years, placing the core hospital specialties at the top, and relegating family medicine, geriatrics and psychiatry to lower positions. The implications of both inter- and intra-professional relationships for the changing pattern of health care, and the drive for economy in provision, are obvious. Adaptation to new work and sensitive allocation of changed roles, the creation of care teams and the development of inter-professional working are all difficult within the current framework and culture. Movement of resources from the hospital to other sectors of care to assist these substantive changes is equally difficult (ibid.).

This latter difficulty is especially significant in view of the growing proportion of the national income, or of government expenditure, absorbed by health care, fuelled by a tradition which has seen such growth as an acceptable feature of public and private finance. Such confident expectation of increasing government support for health care has been undermined by a number of factors. One has been the absolute volume of resources involved and the recent tendency of many governments to seek ways to reduce their public borrowing by reducing public expenditure. Another has been the growing competition for such public expenditure where health has had to argue its case for resources against the claims of an extended array of public services some of which, such as social security, are less easy for governments to control. In those countries where more of the funding for health care is derived directly from individuals or from company-based insurances, the situation is no better as both seek to reduce this area of expenditure, given their increasing costs on other fronts. More importantly, the demographic changes discussed earlier present a pattern of future demand for health care from an ageing population which promises to overshadow anything which has gone before unless the health care available, and popular expectations about that availability, and how it is to be funded, can be changed. There are now grave doubts as to whether the public tax-based purse can afford future care, and the insurance cost of health cover is mounting for individuals as the implications of much greater longevity are reflected in premium rates. Together, these various factors are producing an overwhelming case for changes in the health care system.

CURRENT CHARACTER OF HEALTH CARE SYSTEMS

The changes in the demand for health care and the resources deemed available to meet that demand have to be matched together by health care systems which have developed clear and settled characteristics in their resourcing, organisation and operation. These are worth considering in some detail as they affect very directly any proposals for change in health care, but also have wider significance in relation to professional health care education. Health care systems of course vary in the particular arrangements which they have established, though all tend to show similar tendencies towards professional influence, and there are signs that economic pressures are producing greater convergence. Tables 1.1 and 1.2 show the figures for spending on health care in relation to their Gross Domestic Product for a number of countries, and the division of that spending between public and private sources. Table 1.1 confirms the convergence which is reflected in the broad similarity in national levels of spending on health care although the United States has clearly moved ahead and is spending a good deal more than its European counterparts. These figures also provide some initial evidence of the slowing down of growth in some highly developed systems such as Sweden and the Netherlands. Table 1.2 illustrates the extent to which the level of spending in the United States is driven by private expenditure, but shows the state contribution growing as health care for the poor is developed. The European figures illustrate why governments have become concerned about the impact of growing demand on systems which are so heavily publicly funded. The figures for state spending in 1995 reflect that concern and suggest that the new thinking about public spending and the role of state health care was beginning to impact in most of these cases. The contrast with the United States, with its continued growth in the public sector contribution to spending on health care, reflects its different traditions of social welfare but does suggest that the probable future balance between sectors of expenditure lies somewhere between the United States and the more extreme European models. It is not clear where that balance will eventually fall, but the privatisation of parts of health care in most European countries seems highly likely, while the United States seems likely to develop a more extensive publicly funded health care service.

Table 1.1 *Expenditure on health care as a proportion of GDP, 1960–92*

	1960	1970	1980	1987	1992
Australia	4.6	5.0	6.5	7.1	8.2
Italy	3.3	4.8	6.8	6.9	9.1
Netherlands	3.9	6.0	8.2	8.6	8.9
Sweden	4.7	7.2	9.5	9.0	7.9
UK	3.9	4.5	5.8	6.1	7.5
USA	5.2	7.4	9.2	11.2	13.0

Source: Wall (1996)

Table 1.2 *Public expenditure as a percentage of total health expenditure, 1960–95*

	1960	1970	1975	1980	1985	1995
Australia	48	57	73	63	72	69
Italy	83	86	86	81	77	76
Netherlands	33	84	73	75	75	73
Sweden	73	86	90	93	90	88
UK	85	87	91	90	86	85
USA	25	37	41	42	41	49

Source: Wall (1996)

These patterns of overall spending on health care are important, but more important in relation to our concerns is the more detailed use made of resources and the implications that has for the professions involved and for their education. The long-standing division of developed health care services into clear sectors and the relative importance of those sectors reflected in their share of overall resources, and in other ways, dictate much professional practice and training. Such historical patterns are important and are heavily institutionalised into the existing systems of health care, but they need to be seen increasingly in relation to the economic pressures on health care which are causing necessary changes to be made. Terminology varies between different countries, and the content of work included within sectors also varies, but the broad general distinction between primary, or community-based care, and secondary/tertiary, or hospital-based care, provides the core for our analysis. The hallmark of the developed systems is that both sectors are developed, but the key to understanding the pressure for reform, and the constraints and opportunities conditioning development, lies in the details of the division between them.

Given the overriding importance of economic factors in much current thinking about health care, the distribution of spending between sectors showing the strong emphasis in developed systems on secondary/tertiary care, or to avoid definitional problems, on hospital care, is most significant. Britain offers a clear example of this tendency. Some 60 per cent of public spending within the NHS is devoted to the hospital sector, compared with 40 per cent spent on 'community-based' health care, with only about half of that being spent on the medical aspects of community-based care provided by general practice. Care needs to be taken in making broad aggregate comparisons between sectors, but examination of the pattern of use of the two sectors suggests a *prima facie* case that there may be a tendency for the relationship between the overall demand for care and the allocation of resources to be tilted in favour of the hospitals. In purely medical terms general practice deals with most people's interactions with the health service, and other non-medical community services account for another large tranche of activity (Boaden 1997). It can be argued that many of these interventions are trivial in character, but many are not, and it is in these settings that attitudes towards, and use of, health care services are developed. This is formalised in the central role played by general practice in gatekeeping access to hospital care, helping to manage the flow of demand and screening out intermediate work which might otherwise overwhelm the hospital system. In contrast, hospitals see many fewer cases per year, and most of us experience hospital treatment only infrequently during our lives. Of course the complexity of cases and the character of the treatment given in hospital mean that the unit cost is very high, but even with that proviso, the balance seems inappropriate. Certainly, if chronic care received the attention which it theoretically might do within the system, then the community-based overload would be very significant.

If there is a case for seeing community-based health care as relatively disadvantaged by comparison with hospital care, there are other disparities in both sectors which have direct implications for professional education and training. Comment was made earlier about the hierarchy of specialities within hospital practice, reflecting both the emphasis of current practice and the patterns of influence which have developed within the profession. Such a hierarchy acts to inhibit the movement of resources into emerging specialties and can lead to established interests acting to defend the status quo even when it clearly needs to change. It also affects the development of new specialties because formal status as an independent specialty places activity within the hierarchy in a clearer way allowing for a more transparent allocation of resources. This has other consequences in that the search for such status leads to the growth of more and more specialised areas of care leading to a fragmentation of activity and a concentration on the most highly specialised areas of practice. This in turn promotes a demand for initial education which meets such specialised career needs and leads to early experience being modified by such specialisation.

The powerful impact of such an established hierarchy in both the structure of health care and within the profession is reinforced by the traditions of incremental resource allocation and professional autonomy within education and training. Together they maintain the patterns of relative dominance and force a model of development onto emergent sub-specialities and emergent other professions. Efforts over the years to change the established patterns have proved difficult and confirm the distribution of influence within the profession and the difficulty of reform where established services may have to be changed in order to fund new ones. If the tradition of incremental overall funding in the past did not create opportunities for spending to be re-distributed, it is unlikely to prove easy in the modern context where spending is often declining in real terms. This pattern within hospital specialties also applies to the relationship between hospital and community practice. It seems far more likely that services such as those in the community which were provided cheaply in the past, will be seen as able to provide much more economic ways to extend care in the future by transfer of work from other sectors.

Another dimension of disparity in health care is the geography of provision, and here the inequality relates to spending in both sectors of health care provision. In the case of hospitals, teaching hospitals within the British system have always enjoyed considerable resource advantage, though their wider geographical remit in terms of some specialist care means that the significance of their geographical location is modified. Many are located in inner city areas but this apparent relative accessibility to those in high need of health care may not always materialise. It is particularly significant that conspicuous hospital spending should occur in inner cities because they are the areas within community care which have long been recognised as relatively disadvantaged along with some suburban municipal housing areas (Birch and Maynard 1987). Despite continued efforts at reform, and direct attempts to tackle such inequalities, significant disparities in the provision of health remain across these various dimensions to make Hart's 'Inverse Care Law' as relevant in the late 1990s as it was in the 1970s when he first formulated it (Hart 1971).

It is not easy to extend this discussion from issues of resourcing into consideration of more direct features of health care systems because detailed information about treatment and treatment outcomes is hard to acquire. Starfield has, however, undertaken some analysis of primary medical care in 10 developed countries relating the significance of primary care within their health care system to a satisfaction/expense ratio for such care in each country, and their relative placing in relation to a number of indices of health. Table 1.3, drawn from Starfield, shows the diverse pattern of emphasis on primary care within these 10 health care systems ranging from a score of 0.2 in the United States to 1.7 in the United Kingdom (Starfield 1992). The UK's highest score in terms of primary care emphasis is consistent with the reputation of

Table 1.3 *Primary care scores, satisfaction/expense index and health indicators for 10 industrialised countries*

	Primary care score	Satisfaction expense index	Health indicators	
			Top third	Bottom third
Australia	1.1	2.1	3	0
Belgium	0.8	NA	0	9
Canada	1.2	7.6	5	0
Denmark	1.5	NA	0	3
Finland	1.5	NA	5	6
Germany (FR)	0.5	2.9	1	7
Netherlands	1.5	9.0	10	0
Sweden	1.2	4.3	10	0
United Kingdom	1.7	2.1	0	8
United States	0.2	0.2	1	7

Source: Starfield (1992, p. 230)

British primary care, although a number of recent reforms are changing the nature of that primary care and may be reducing that overall score. The value of that high score, and the significance of primary care in relation to the health of the public are put into perspective, however, when indices of health are considered, at any rate on the comparative basis employed here. The United Kingdom does badly on this measure, raising a number of questions about the significance of the emphasis given to primary care. As Starfield is at pains to point out, health is a complex indicator and one has to examine many factors outside the formal health care system in order to explain why some countries do well and others less well. She points clearly to the lack of government spending in relation to areas like social security, good housing and education, widely regarded as causally related to health conditions, as being more significant for health indices. Primary care may be significant in mitigating the effects of shortfalls in these other areas, but that opens up a significant area of alternative debate about the wider role which primary, or community care, might take. The character of primary care and its geographical distribution becomes the issue, as does its relationship with other relevant factors in other sectors, both public and private, which influence the state of public health. Ultimately there are questions to be addressed about the quality and character of primary care being offered and whether more impact could be obtained with current resource levels but with some reform of their use. It is interesting for our later discussion that primary care in the United Kingdom only scores modestly in terms of community orientation (Starfield 1992).

Despite the lack of firm evidence about some of these issues, there seems to be a general tendency in the developed world to advocate a shift of health care emphasis from hospital care into the community. Two sorts of argument support this emphasis. One is the financial case just discussed. It is clear that primary care provides large sections of the community with their main access to health care, and that it does so at very modest overall, and unit, cost. Of course much of that care is trivial, some of it probably even unnecessary in strict medical terms, but it is the sector where care is accessible, and where potentially serious conditions can be first diagnosed and access to hospital care sensibly managed. It is also a setting in which more direct care might be provided, inhibiting the flow of demand for more expensive care delivery in hospitals. It may even be that functions now undertaken in hospitals could be undertaken within primary care, changing the nature of professional activity there in significant ways. Undertaking more care in the community in all of these ways is an appealing option for governments, although two caveats should be borne in mind.

The volume of care provided in the primary setting already imposes considerable pressure on available medical resources and an escalation in use will involve significant changes in professional and associated staff practice, or an increase in the numbers of staff involved, or some combination of such changes. More can be done, and the quality of what is done can be improved but not without significant change. Both are important contributions if the benefits of a shift in the emphasis of health care into the community are to achieve its goals. It seems likely that spending in the sector will have to increase, and there is always a risk that change could simply involve a dilution in the quality of care. More economic forms of provision are certainly possible, but standards of effectiveness must be maintained if measures of cost-effectiveness become established as the criteria for evaluating future community-based health care.

This issue is bound up with the intention of many reformers that the changes must be much more than a simple extension of conventional primary care. They envisage a considerable movement of work currently undertaken in expensive hospital settings into the community. This involves the offering of some minor treatments in primary care, but also the movement of most treatment after-care out of the hospital. Short-stay treatments and day-care provision are two of the most obvious developments already occurring in hospitals to limit the non-clinical costs of care and maximise the use of expensive staff and equipment. The implications of such changes for primary care need to be anticipated and decisions taken about how they will be met if they are not to result in future unplanned consequences for patients and for the health services.

This debate about the balance between hospital and community care in the treatment of acute conditions raises the fundamental question about sectors of care and the proper medical justification for care being undertaken in one sector or another. It is clear that there are cases at each end of the spectrum of care which clearly belong where they are. Trivial conditions may not even require attention, but if they do, then the community setting is where that is best offered and most accessible. In contrast are the conditions of acute medical need where the hospital is currently the only setting in which tests and procedures can be made available in a controlled context and with the benefit of the extensive ancillary resources needed. In between are a wide range of conditions, some of which have gone into one sector while others have gone into another. Extensive debates about the quality of referrals to hospital from the community, and about self-referral to Accident and Emergency Departments reveal the implications of decisions within the grey area and illustrate the impact of inadequate inter-sectoral relationships, or of direct patient demand. A more appropriate distribution of this workload, and a more self-conscious management of professional workloads could yield financial benefits, without consequent loss in the quality of medical care provided.

It is worth considering the arguments for increased community-based provision. These rest on a number of factors, some related to the patients involved and some to the character of the medical care which is possible in that context. In terms of patients, community-based care allows them to be treated in their normal surroundings, with continuing access to informal care and support networks. It allows normal living to continue within the constraints imposed by the medical condition, and provides a patient-friendly basis for treatment which takes into account the features of normal life.

These are the characteristics which have always underpinned community-based health care around the management of chronic illness and episodes of acute ill-health of a minor kind. This traditional emphasis remains a central focus of community-based health care, but the policy arguments in health are promoting a wider discussion about who should undertake such work. Movement of more acute work into the community reinforces the need to consider who does what in the context of community-based health care. Treatment may be provided differently and there are clear options for cheaper, but equally effective, members of the primary health care team to undertake some of the more traditional work. Community-based work allows the division of labour between the doctor and other semi-professional primary care staff to be considered more rationally and more coherently.

More important perhaps is the discussion about community-based care which extends the debate even more widely beyond the realms of the traditional professional concern with direct medical care. This embraces the concept of population-based medicine and what is normally termed a public health perspective. It recognises the complex relationship between the wide-ranging causes of ill health and addresses the relationships between doctors in the community and a wide range of other agencies and organisations who operate within that setting and whose activities do influence people's health. Such concerns do arise within the traditional notion of care and are central to the role of primary care in providing continuity and comprehensiveness of care. They assume a wider significance if the decision is taken to move away from the traditional idea of medicine as narrowly focused on treating individual patients.

The spread of options involved in community-based health care amply justifies the concerted efforts being made to promote such emphases on both economic and clinical grounds. In themselves these have longer-term implications for traditional medical education. The increasing specialisation of much hospital treatment and the high cost involved are limiting the ability to use the hospitals as a site for basic medical education in the traditional way. The extent of student knowledge and the experience of applying clinical skills are seriously limited. Movement of care into the community, and the extent of existing community practice mean that this requirement can be met outside the hospitals, but in addition the other challenges posed by community practice itself must also be addressed.

2

Traditional medical education

Chapter 1 outlined some of the heavy demands facing the health care systems of most developed countries and the increasing emphasis being placed on community-based health care as a result. In turn these changes in health care are giving rise to widespread discussion about needed changes in health care education if the character and mix of professional staff are not to become even further out of line with the services they provide. A number of important developments in medical education have already emerged in different countries over recent years, reflecting recognition of the need for change, and the stage of thinking about the kinds of changes which are required. Before examining those developments in more detail it is important to describe the long-standing model of medical education which is being changed, but which remains widespread in practice.

In fact, medical education has enjoyed a relatively stable pattern over a long period of time providing perhaps the best example of the generic, ideal–typical model of professional education and training. This does not mean that reform, or efforts at reform, are a recent phenomenon. In an overview of past reform initiatives in medical education in the United States, Enarsun and Burg review 15 major studies undertaken between 1904 and 1992, revealing continuing concern about some basic issues but quite modest levels of change and development, pointing up the complexity of a reform process where 'All stakeholder groups involved in medical education will need to work together to develop a national database that facilitates critical analysis and improvements in the entire medical education process – education, evaluation, accreditation, certification and licensure' (Enarsun and Burg 1992, p. 1141). In the United Kingdom the efforts date back to an even earlier period, and the limits on successful reform reflect the same institutional barriers and the prevailing attitudes among the key stakeholders in medical education. Professional control of the educational process has not proved a model capable of responding to the dynamic demands of the changing health care context.

THE BASIC MODEL

This pattern of relative inertia, or at best reform by modest curriculum extension to embrace additions to the traditional core, is typical of much professional education. Professional status, for medicine as for other established professions, allows high levels of autonomy to the individual doctor in his or her practice. This autonomy, startlingly different from the position of the health care occupations who have not successfully professionalised, is legitimised by the medical profession exercising control over recruitment to, training for, and discipline among its members. This guarantees acceptable standards of autonomous practice and the profession undertakes to discipline, and if necessary remove from practice, any member who falls short of those acceptable standards of practice. The exercise of these controls and the maintenance of public confidence rest on a number of features of professional practice and consequently of professional education.

First and foremost is the presence of a core basic academic discipline which forms the knowledge base which underpins professional practice. In the case of medicine, the nature of practice means that this disciplinary base is accompanied by a range of practical skills, mastery of which is deemed essential to competent professional performance. Together this combination of knowledge and skills constitute the character of the professional role, and acquisition of both guarantees the quality of professional work. The character and quality of professional practice are further guaranteed by the establishment of appropriate professional attitudes and values which are legitimised through the formally established ethical codes which medicine has adopted to govern appropriate practice. The guarantee of these three interlocking characteristics, knowledge, skills and attitude, underlies public acceptance of professional status and autonomy, and the profession has created a range of institutions which act to ensure that registered members possess and maintain them.

In order to establish these three key professional characteristics, and to induct new members into appropriate practice, the profession has developed an elaborate system of education and training. This itself displays a number of important characteristics. First, in keeping with the claims made about necessary knowledge, skills and attitudes to be established prior to professional accreditation, is a very long period of initial education. In formal terms this involves 5 years in medical school, followed by a year's experience of practice before formal registration as an accredited doctor. Beyond this there is further postgraduate training and supervised experience before the doctor can enter his or her chosen specialty as a fully autonomous practitioner. In the nature of medical practice both knowledge and skills will change, and both may raise new ethical challenges for doctors in practice so that, despite this very long induction, there remains a need for continuing medical education throughout the career. Formally, however, this is much less developed than initial training, posing sharp challenges to the long-term legitimacy of some professional practice, particularly in volatile health care situations such as those discussed in Chapter 1.

Returning to the initial period of education and training, a number of features of the process are worthy of comment. One feature is the knowledge base which underpins the work done in medical school. The biological sciences have provided that base for a long time and the bio-medical model of illness and treatment provides the intellectual and methodological base for professional practice. This emphasis is reflected in recruitment into medical school where the conventional requirement is to have studied science to a level from which medical school can continue the linear development of higher level knowledge and skills. This narrow approach is entirely consistent with the establishment of a legitimate sphere of professional practice, and it should be said, is consistent with the models of practice adopted widely within the hospital setting. Its utility in some other health care settings may be open to more challenge and the development of training for community-based practice suggests that the character of such practice is significantly different.

Of course concentration on bio-medical issues does not mean that the content of professional syllabuses remains unchanged. The biological sciences have expanded substantially and have fragmented into ever more highly specialised areas, posing a considerable challenge to those responsible for medical education. This expansion of the traditional core knowledge can overload the curriculum even before account has been taken of the wider development of health care which makes other disciplines relevant to our understanding of disease, but more importantly to our understanding of treatment and action to prevent disease or promote better health. This widening of the proper concerns of intending doctors poses two challenges. One, often repeated over the years when reform has been considered, is the sheer volume of material involved in mastering the range of disciplines adequately. The other, less often the subject of debate, is the philosophy and methodology of science which apply to the core areas of medicine, but which become more attenuated as the range of disciplines extends to accommodate wider approaches to health and health care. Sociology and some areas of psychology are far removed in their approach from biology and chemistry, raising difficulties in the recruitment phase of professional education, but also in the character of teaching and learning involved in initial professional education. A narrowly scientific view can lead to the rejection of evidence, and of attitudes, which are central to the understanding and treatment of many contemporary diseases, and it can lead to serious inter-professional problems where doctors and others drawing on different disciplines meet to provide multi-professional care.

Other issues arise from these characteristics because they have created a traditional educational model within medical school which has two major elements. One arose from the very large body of material which had to be covered and which created a preference for highly didactic teaching methods and an emphasis on systematic learning associated with frequent tests of knowledge applied as the dominant method of student assessment. The other was the establishment of an apprentice system in relation to the acquisition of skills and the inculcation of professional values in which an experienced doctor became the guide and mentor to the medical student and the junior doctor. The didactic, teacher-centred character of both these aspects of medical education secured high levels of competence in terms of the knowledge and skill base of practice, and strong compliance with the established professional attitudes. These should not be dismissed lightly nor should the methods which give rise to such successful outcomes. There are, however, other more negative implications. One is the danger of new doctors modelling their behaviour and practice on less than adequate role models, particularly in a context where such role models see teaching as only a minor aspect of their role. The other is that the didactic teaching model may not be the best preparation for a career of continuing personal and professional development which relies on a high level of self-direction. Nor for a career in which the pace of change in both the range and content of the science involved, and in the organisation of health care, is extremely rapid. The movement of more health care into the community, as discussed in Chapter 1, certainly makes the current knowledge base and role models of less utility than they were for traditional practice within the hospital setting.

Such generic initial education and training provide the core elements which support professional status, but developments in medicine and the increasing complexity of health care mean that most doctors are involved in further education and development in shaping their specialisation within the profession. This post-qualifying specialist training is of shorter duration, and is much looser and less formal in character, varying with the specialty and with the career progression of the individual. Looking back at the character of initial education, this postgraduate phase continues the change of emphasis evident in the later years of medical school. Formal teaching becomes relatively marginal as the basic science has been mastered, and supervised practical experience, even if supervision is sometimes nominal, continues the apprenticeship model. Following this postgraduate training, the subsequent career within the chosen specialty involves only a modest input of formal continuing professional education despite the fact that it may cover thirty years of practice, and considerable change in that practice. This limitation on further formal education and training results from the resource implications for doctors engaged fully in health care delivery. The professional need to maintain currency in practice and keep up to date with developments is left to the individual doctor who is expected to maintain his or her own development. This structure places a heavy burden on initial training. It is expected to provide the substantive base for a long career, possibly in quite varied specialties. It is also expected to develop the intellectual and organisational capacities, and the motivation, which are necessary to sustain and adjust individual practice over career-long continuing professional development.

A further aspect of this model is that the setting for most medical education and training tends to be the context where the dominant aspects of training can most readily be applied. This has meant that most medical education, certainly in terms of the experience needed for skills development, has been undertaken in the hospital setting. This is where the science is most obviously relevant, and where there is a high concentration of seriously ill patients who provide the raw material on which to test the science and hone the emergent skills of medical practice. It is also the place in which to observe the dominant role models in the profession, and to absorb the conventions of practice in relation to colleagues, other staff, and of course, patients. Less desirably perhaps, it is also where students become aware of the patterns of professional dominance reflected in different specialties, in individual status, and in the patterns of resource allocation which reflect those factors. Choice of specialty and attitudes towards other specialties are developed during this phase of professional development and can have significant effects on future multi-disciplinary work.

The other characteristic of this system which is important here is that it is essentially controlled and managed by the profession itself. Several things flow from this. First, the maintenance of that professional autonomy depends on the presence of a publicly acceptable system for assessing new entrants to the profession, accrediting their professional training and guaranteeing their competence to practice. This is evident in the formal system of accreditation and in the extended period of supervised experience, culminating in early hospital practice which continues to be subject to professional scrutiny. Practice in the community is much less readily scrutinised and independent practice may be taken on much sooner than in the hospital. Second is a conservatism, partly justified by the wish to maintain public confidence, and so professional control, both of which might be seen as threatened by any programme of radical change. This conservatism also arises from the fact that education and training reflect the dominant patterns of attitude and influence within the profession and, given a degree of institutional inertia within the profession, this is often a long-established and so, possibly, outmoded pattern. In some respects this is a model which best represents yesterday's practice, may be able to deal with today's, but finds tomorrow's practice difficult to introduce into the overcrowded curriculum.

Postgraduate training and education go some way towards addressing that criticism. All areas of medicine involve a period of postgraduate training, and continuing supervision by an established specialist. This will involve exposure to current professional practice and to a number of specialties in order to give the new doctor a range of experience. Some specialties provide more opportunity than others, of course, and newly emerging specialties such as virology or palliative care, may be more difficult to establish on this model. This affects the choice of specialty among new entrants, especially when the experience of medical school will have predisposed many students to a choice of specialism already. This is evident in the United States where medical schools are struggling to orientate more students towards careers in community-based practice. This is not a problem in the United Kingdom, where there are enough entrants choosing this option, though it is interesting that their subsequent formal postgraduate training for general practice involves a year's exposure to that specialty, but also two further years spent in hospital specialties deemed to be relevant to the work of a general practitioner. The service needs of hospitals dictate this pattern, resulting in a continuing emphasis on the hospital sector even within community-oriented education.

For most purposes this period of postgraduate education is experiential in character with a minimum of academic material and formal instruction and a high premium placed on direct experience of patient consultations and treatment. In this sense it represents a continuation of earlier training and reflects the fact that such training is very general in character and is only a preparation for the concentration involved in preparing to specialise. This makes the balance between the two parts an interesting issue and does raise questions about the nature and length of the initial period when compared with the later. This is particularly important when the emphasis moves to community-based practice. The demand for 5 years vocational training to make the transition into the community reflects the reality of hospital demands rather than the needs of community practice.

Once formal professional training is complete, the specialist doctor, whether in hospital or the community, is subject to expectations in relation to continuing education, but to very modest formal requirements. A few hours each year of formal attendance at educational sessions is the limit of the requirement. A major explanation for the limit is the complexity of releasing doctors for more attendance given their central role in health care delivery. A different explanation lies in the absence of any developed system to cater for their needs throughout a lengthy career of changing practice. These two constraints combine to limit discussion about continuing education, although general practice in the United Kingdom, with its own more developed rules, has begun to establish a more elaborate approach.

It is worth dwelling on this latter development which is beginning to distinguish between continuing medical education, continuing professional development, and continuing personal development as three distinct aspects of the process. All are important in a career which involves high levels of patient contact and which demands difficult judgements on expensive and complex ethical issues. Medical school in theory should have provided the groundwork for all of these, but it is clear that the early emphasis in professional training emphasises medical education. Professional training too is dominated by clinical concerns, leaving professional and personal development to be dealt with in continuing education, which is limited in scope and scale. In the absence of more developed formal systems of education, these key areas of professional and personal growth are left to the individual to handle within their practice using whatever diverse resources are available. The fact that practice may be changing in radical ways makes this challenge all the more difficult.

EDUCATION FOR EXISTING COMMUNITY ROLES

This traditional model is very heavily based on a career which leads through the hospital hierarchy towards a consultant post in a chosen specialty. In such a professional climate there was a time when any other career path in medicine was conceived by many as a sign of failure, and the disdain for community-based practice was reflected in its limited place in relation to education and training. This is especially significant now as health care systems begin to emphasise community-based practice as more central to overall health care and as a consequence seek to have more resources used within the community. The medical school curriculum was not designed with such community-based practice in mind, but the view taken of such practice within the profession led to the assumption being made that it was a perfectly adequate preparation in any case. Such views were challenged in the post-war period with the development of general practice with its own College of General Practitioners analogous to other specialties and the subsequent development of compulsory postgraduate education particular to that specialty. This challenge has grown with the development of that system which has involved an implicit, and in some circumstances explicit, critique of initial medical education, at least as a preparation for community-based practice. This has involved issues of content and of attitudes and values, but more importantly has incorporated a different approach in the educational processes deemed appropriate for professional training for such practice.

The development of this system has important implications for any further development of community-based practice. As the current model of community-based education within professional medicine it may too easily be taken as the model for future development and as providing a model for the development of a community-oriented undergraduate medical curriculum. Such a transfer requires much wider discussion, both of current experience and of future need. As was commented earlier the structure of postgraduate vocational training for general practice is by no means what the Royal College of General Practitioners would have wished when the system was first introduced. They failed in their bid for 5 years of postgraduate training which would have aligned general practice with hospital specialties. They also failed to obtain more than 1 year of direct experience within general practice during the 3 years of full training which were approved. Registrars preparing for general practice play an important role in the delivery of hospital-based services and these cannot be put at risk in the interests of training for community roles, reflecting the traditional dominance of the hospital sector and the difficulty of coping with the resource implications of change. More positively, those hospital experiences do reflect the fact that a key role within community-based medicine involves managing the interface with hospital care, making experience within hospitals more relevant than would otherwise be the case. No doubt it also reflects the view that the clinical aspects of general practice, because of their generality, can be dealt with adequately with the basic knowledge and skills acquired in medical school. In short, it is not a specialty in the way that hospital specialties are. The elements that make it special fall outside the core bio-medical curriculum.

In a sense this is correct in relation to much practice which lies at the core of community-based medicine. It is the extensions from that core involved in such practice which then become most interesting. These include the following:

- a more holistic approach to the patient;
- a more contextual approach to the patient;
- a more continuing approach to the patient;
- a more comprehensive approach to the patient;
- a more preventive approach to the patient.

These extensions have led to a claim for general practice as being quite distinct from hospital practice. Despite such claims, development has led to a model of medical education in general practice which is in some respects quite like the traditional hospital model, different only in that it is learned within the community-based surgery rather than the hospital ward. The obvious similarity is the high emphasis placed on experiential learning under the supervision of an existing practitioner. This occupies the year in general practice and is conceived as providing the basis for a steady evolution from modest, supervised practice, to a situation where the Registrar manifests readiness for independent practice by carrying something close to a conventional clinic workload. This rapid movement towards independent practice contrasts with the hospital approach and is a significant aspect of the change of attitudes and the acquisition of new core skills intended to reflect the difference between doctor–patient interactions in the community and those in hospital. As with hospital training, so in general practice, supervision is the key element in this system. Unlike the hospital system, however, general practice has recognised the change involved in practising in the community and so been much more self-conscious about the educational processes involved. An elaborate system has been developed to accredit and manage a large group of GP Trainers who provide the one-to-one supervision required by the system. These Trainers are themselves trained for this role, unlike their hospital counterparts, and are expected to develop some special capacities in relation to their teaching role, rather than it being a mere extension of their practice. This followed an earlier period when the selection of GPs known to be good doctors, and assumed therefore to be good teachers, demonstrated that this assumption was misplaced (Horder and Swift 1979).

It is in the context of this different model of education that some of the new elements in medical education have emerged which are now being applied more widely. Education for general practice in establishing the claim to be a separate specialty has been involved in an implicit, and sometimes explicit, critique of medical school education. The result has been a search for educational models deemed more appropriate to community-based practice. It has found these in the theory and practice of adult education, valued for itself in relation to the processes involved, but also an approach to education which in part mirrors the professional view of the ideal–typical doctor–patient relationship in the community setting. This approach tightly links the character of medical education and medical practice, at least in terms of a particular model of that practice.

Despite these claims, and 20 years of consolidation of this system, it remains uncertain as to how far education and training for general practice have succeeded in their aims. The nature of both training and practice makes evidence about the process and thus about its quality difficult to acquire. There is, however, some evidence that entrants into general practice often regard their training as having been an inadequate preparation for practice. This is often a reflection of issues which the model of training does not address rather than the inadequacy of the training for those which it does. Many of these are the wider contextual issues within which face-to-face consultations take place, and which are a key aspect of those extensions of role outlined earlier as characteristic of community-based practice. The other feature of this system is that, despite the philosophy which underpins practice, it seems not to provide the capacity for continuing self-directed learning necessary in a volatile health service. Adaptation to change, the ability to manage evidence-based practice and the capacity to work with emerging new professional groups are not obvious features of professional reaction to change. The strong resistance to changes in practice is partly a result of how those changes have been introduced, but also arises from a professional difficulty in coping with change. This poses a serious challenge to a future which, as was outlined in Chapter 1, seems likely to involve more rather than less change.

THE MOVEMENT FOR CHANGE

For some considerable time there have been moves afoot to change the educational system outlined above. Some of the arguments used reflect the earlier discussion about changes in health care, but many take up what has been a long-standing debate within the profession. For professionals seeking to promote change it is useful to invoke the issues concerning the relationship between education and care, but the debate quickly reverts to questions relating to adaptation of the existing system. The important paper from the GMC in Britain looking at the character of future doctors, spells out the failures of past reform efforts and the character of the debate, recalling in particular several past reports which advocated a reduction in the factual content of medical education and a broadening of its intellectual base (General Medical Council 1993). It is not the intention here to rehearse the issues which have hindered past efforts at reform. Suffice it to say that they reflect the professional context in which they arose, a long period in which the profession exercised a limiting influence on health care reform and with it, a conservative view about appropriate medical education. This is neatly summarised in relation to the United States where it is asserted that 'The medical profession . . . has historically demonstrated an uncanny knack for asserting what the sociologist Paul Starr has termed its "sovereignty" over both the clinical practice and the business of medicine' (Grumbach 1995).

Two strands of educational reform may be distinguished and can be related to quite different aspects of changes in the context of health care, although it is not clear that they are motivated by concerns for that relationship. One arises from the changing context of health care provision and the shift from a hospital-based towards a more community-based orientation. The other arises from the changing nature of health care and the limitations on the degree to which formal continuing education can meet the demands implicit in change. This has led to a recognition of the need to equip doctors more effectively for a lifetime of continuing professional development and so avoid the difficulties which have arisen in the past over change and adaptation.

The first of these has tended towards the view that education for general practice may provide a model worth adopting more widely for doctors in training. In some countries this takes the form that experience in the community may encourage recruitment to community practice. In others it is more an issue of seeking to share the values and approach inherent in current community-based education.

The second is much more complex. It posits the view that if the nature of continuing professional development involves a high degree of reflective practice and self-directed learning, partly because of the absence of more formal educational opportunities, then it is necessary to provide trainee doctors with an educational base that will lead to the development of the necessary learning skills to manage that development. This is the approach being advocated in British general practice, and in some of the earlier innovations in medical schools, all of them tracing their roots into various strands of adult education theory which emerged strongly in the 1970s (Brookfield 1986).

It is worth distinguishing some of these antecedents here. They reflect the work of a number of educational theorists concerned with a range of issues related to the characteristics of adults as learners, and in consequence, the type of teaching and learning needed for their exploitation. Summarising a number of formulations they involve the following:

1 The adult learner as someone who has reached a maturity which allows movement away from dependency in many aspects of life, creating a capacity for self-direction which is then reflected as a preferred learning style. The contrast with the style of traditional medical education could hardly be more marked.
2 The adult learner is, by definition, someone with experience and that experience can and should be converted into an effective learning resource, although care may be needed in translating this general concept into the context of professional education.
3 The adult learner is motivated to learn by features of their own development and by the changing roles which are experienced in maturity. This generalised concept

can readily be translated into the professional medical context though care needs to be exercised in relation to the character of professional development.

4 The adult learner is someone whose orientation to learning is moving away from a subject orientation towards a concern with problems and their solution. The contrast with the traditional approach of medical schools outlined earlier could not be more sharp.

(Knowles 1970)

The changes needed in medical education to accommodate this learning model are evident, although it does possess features which reflect the heavy emphasis on experience within traditional medical education in its later stages. The corollary of these characteristics of the adult learner is a need for the organisation and style of the educational process to be adjusted to take account of the developmental change from the old didactic system towards this new learner-centred approach. Teaching in the traditional didactic mode may be inappropriate to such adult learners, though there will remain situations in which it remains a part of the education of a trainee professional. At the same time other methods will be appropriate to later stages of that education. The key to success lies in the creation of an educational system which recognises the challenge involved in, and the stages necessary, to move from the traditional approach to an approach which is more sensitive to students and their needs (Grow 1991).

THE MOVEMENT TOWARDS REFORM

For some years now the varied pressures discussed above have led to a movement for reform in medical education which has slowly gathered momentum. Inevitably perhaps, in a context where medical education has been slow to respond to changes in medicine and medical care, the scale of reform needed to bring education into line, let alone begin to prepare for the future, is very great. This assumes added significance in a professional context where such radicalism has serious implications for the profession and its established order, but where continuing professional control may be removed if the profession cannot itself make significant moves towards reform.

Reform is made more complicated by the range of demands which the new medical education has to meet. In terms of health care provision there is the clear move to more care being provided in the community rather than in hospital. This in turn has serious consequences for professional roles in both settings, with significant shifts of professional influence from the hospital specialities towards the community. This is made more difficult by the traditional view taken within the profession about the two types of medical role, partly fuelled by the fact that community roles bring the wider issues of new disciplines and new orientations into play. A third pressure comes from the need within the profession to provide adequate guarantees about career-long practice with wide implications for continuing education and for the base on which it needs to build. The new education must serve all these demands.

The result has been a range of experiments with change, mainly within the undergraduate curriculum, but some aimed at the later stages of professional education and training. The pattern of change and the disproportionate effort going into undergraduate teaching and learning reflect the traditional dominance of early professional education, with little attention being paid to more radical possibilities in relation to the balance of time spent in the different stages of medical education. The argument continues to be the traditional one that if early education is of a good standard, then it can provide the base for lifelong learning and other aspects of medical education will be adjusted to meet the needs which emerge.

It is worth clarifying the range of reforms being discussed. In terms of the new orientation of health care, the dominant emphasis lies in the development of community-based education which enjoys parity with the hospital-oriented aspects which have dominated in the past. This comes in a variety of guises, ranging from community-based learning, through community-oriented medical education, to learning within general practice or primary care. These are by no means all the same and it is important to distinguish them conceptually if we are to have a clear discussion and evaluation of these innovations.

Community-based learning is learning undertaken by the medical student in one of many community settings which may range from the GP practice, through the health centre, to any of the various venues in which health care is now being delivered outside the hospital. These will be discussed in greater detail in Chapter 5.

Community-oriented medical education is medical education organised both practically and intellectually around the needs and concerns which arise in communities in relation to their health and health care. It often takes place in the same venues which are used for community-based learning, but need not do so, and can be engaged in the context of traditional classroom-based teaching. Experientially it demands consideration both of where and how it is best undertaken.

Learning within general practice follows the model developed in introducing students and trainees to that specialty, but is constrained by the current character of general practice in terms of what is learned. It need not be constrained in that way, and could be involved with more general medical education, but the model closely resembles the hospital-based tradition with slightly different emphases. Learning within primary care widens the context to provide for student learning within the broader-based primary care team, allowing the development of ideas and approaches which are more limited if it remains within the narrower context of general practice.

This combination of features has led to increased interest in community-based education. This aspect of the drive towards change derives from the patterns of training for primary care roles which have developed over the past 30 years in the postgraduate setting. There has long been a recognition that initial medical education was not a suitable preparation for practice outside hospital and this has led to quite explicit postgraduate training. This should not be exaggerated, however, as we have seen in the British case, it involves only a year spent in general practice, with two further years of relevant hospital experience as well. The latter is problematic in that the direct experience is seen as relevant to general practice but the teaching associated with that practice is widely regarded as not dealing with that relevance in any effective way. The former is more important to our purposes here.

The year spent in general practice is regarded as a re-learning for most doctors. The orientation is different, the nature of the experience is different and the whole approach to practice is different from that experienced in hospital. Patients in all states of health are seen, with many not really ill at all, and some evincing the symptoms of serious illness. The trainee doctor learns to handle a new approach to diagnosis dictated by this cross-sectional patient group. It is no longer a search for confirmation of a disease pre-diagnosed on referral, but rather a search for what might be a disease, or might be symptoms which arise from a wide range of factors. It is no longer a decision about standard treatments, but a consideration of cases within their wider context. It is a matter of treating the whole patient, in their family and community setting and learning to take account of those factors in doing so. In many cases it is a matter of dealing with uncertainty in so far as the doctor becomes the first point of contact with a patient. Above all it seems it is necessary to learn a range of skills which were not learned during the passage through medical school in terms of consultation styles and communication skills.

The issue of career-long learning and the need to prepare doctors for that is a more complex one. This is not a matter of where experience is found, and how it is organised, but reflects the whole style of teaching and learning involved in medical school. Once again it is argued that a new approach to learning has developed in the context of community-based practice where the demands just outlined have required a different treatment of the trainee doctor. In effect, the educational approach has come to reflect the style of interaction with patients, echoing the criticism of much medical school education and the way patients were traditionally treated within the hospital setting.

UNDERGRADUATE CURRICULUM REFORM

The changes in health care systems outlined in Chapter 1 have produced significant pressures on the traditional model of professional education. The growing emphasis on primary care in the community has given the models of existing community-based medical education considerable influence, but the overwhelming case for change has been driven by the importance of appropriately trained professional staff to deliver any model of systemic change. The reform movement in education turns on the relationship between health care and health care education and the fact that the former has become more volatile while the latter has remained more stable and is less liable to change. The resulting incongruence between the two raises questions about the survival of the existing educational system, and certainly about the continuing autonomy involved in professional control of that education. If adjustment in education undertaken within the profession falls below the level necessary to deliver satisfactory reform in the health care system, government may have to intervene to influence the educational system more directly.

It is not surprising in such a context that in the United Kingdom it is the Chief Medical Officer in the Department of Health who has been a prime mover in promoting educational reform. In the United States the case is somewhat different, with the insurance companies and systems of managed care making demands for more doctors to opt for community-based careers. The detailed motivations in different countries vary with the characteristics of the health care system but all seem to be producing a demand for reform along now well-established community-based lines.

3

Community-based learning for clinicians

The discussion of community-based practice and education in the earlier chapters reflects very clearly the development of medicine and of medical services in the developed world and stands in sharp contrast to the experience in the developing world. Evidence from many developing countries and from the World Health Organisation (WHO) suggests that they take a different view about the style and purpose of community-based practice and of education for such practice. Both reflect the clear differences between the developed and developing world in terms of the context and character of their health care systems, and, though to a less marked degree, their health care education.

In the developed world, primary care has only recently become central to health care policy, driven by the escalating cost of, and demand for, secondary and tertiary care. In developing countries health care systems have long concentrated on primary care, partly because of their more scattered rural populations, and partly because they have never been able to afford to adopt the models of care of developed countries. Health care education has been less independent of influence from developed countries as professional control has taken on a more global force and the legacy of many educational institutions has been to follow the colonial model in dealing with developing countries. Nevertheless, there has been more pressure for health care education to reflect the realities of health care provision, if only because of the very high cost of adopting Western educational models. This dual pattern of different development is evident in the commitment among developing countries to the Alma Ata Declaration of 1978 and to the World Federation for Medical Education Edinburgh Declaration of 1988 (see pp. 91–2).

In short, it seems that the developing world has had to accept the need for health care and professional education to be much more integrated in ways which are only now becoming apparent in the developed countries. The potential relevance of the developing country experience is evident in much of the rhetoric about necessary change in Europe and the United States and the curriculum innovation in some developing country medical schools may have much to offer those planning change elsewhere.

Before looking at particular examples of curriculum development in such countries, it may be worth examining more closely the philosophy which underpins the approach being adopted. Several aspects may be distinguished, reflecting the complexity discussed earlier, but highlighting those features deemed most relevant to the approach. First is the overriding recognition that there must be integration of education and practice, at all levels and across related sectors. Principle 9 of the Edinburgh Declaration made it clear that co-ordination of medical education and health care delivery was a central requirement for the future. The European follow-up to Edinburgh led to the Lisbon Initiative which spelt out what that meant in formal institutional terms. There was a need for:

> Clear and effective mechanisms should foster close cooperation between the health and education sectors in the establishment of policy and programmes for health professional education.
>
> Education programmes in individual universities and medical schools should reflect the above-mentioned country policies.
>
> *Medical Education* (1996)

The parallel consultation for Africa recommended the more active development of national and regional task forces which could take such policies forward. Such high-level determinations are the essence of international development where complex cross-national groups are seeking consensual outcomes with few existing institutions to give them shape and form. They reflect the *de facto* globalisation of so much of health care and medicine and the absence of international institutions to give it shape, while national institutions tend to assert their differences.

More importantly they reflect a widely shared philosophy about what is required in relation to health care, and as a consequence, in relation to professional education in health care. This is conceived as a new paradigm for the relationship between health institutions and the community moving from:

> paternalism to partnership; from instruction delivery to communication and interaction; from practitioners centred to patient- and people-centred care; from 'curative' to preventive, primitive and rehabilitative; from solitary focused education to a two-way process of community benefit and education gain; from institutional 'isolation' in the

medical field to the wide sphere of inter-sectoral collaboration and community participation.

(Ezzat 1995)

From there Ezzat goes on to spell out the pivotal role of the community in health professions education, and the necessary conditions to give effect to that pivotal role. This is in stark contrast to the ASME (Association for the Study of Medical Education) report which talks of community education as 'any teaching in the undergraduate course that is not hospital based' (*The Lancet* 1994) which is counterposed to a view of learning about the community which involves 'its health status, its organisational units, prevalent medical conditions, self-defined health needs, barriers to meeting those needs, and use of health resources in the community' (ibid.).

As in all such cases the rhetoric of international conferences and the reality of practice on the ground do not necessarily correspond. It is therefore important to look at examples of curriculum development to see what has been attempted and what success has been achieved. The following cases illustrate the diversity of efforts and confirm the wide range of aims and objectives associated with community-based learning.

These examples from very different countries illustrate some common themes but confirm the diversity of approach in what are often seen as uniformly community-oriented developments. They confirm the complexity of the issues involved and the need for much greater clarity when engaging reform in the context of countries where health care systems and professional education are more firmly established.

YAOUNDE, CAMEROON

In this case development of the curriculum occurred as long ago as the mid-1960s following recognition that the Western model of medical education was inappropriate to the health care needs experienced in Cameroon (Monekosso 1993). Development followed two innovatory phases. The first introduced a strong emphasis on public health and the second followed the rejection in 1963 of a WHO proposal for a Western-type medical school. Instead it was recommended that there should be a multi-professional teaching programme which would combine the education of all members of the health care team. In addition, there would be a stress placed on the vertical integration of studies, incorporating elements of primary care and utilising problem-solving as a learning method throughout the 6 years of training. The programme was both community-oriented (emphasising the needs of the community as distinct from those of the individual) and community-based in that learning would take place physically in the community. The aim was to produce doctors who were general duty (omnipractitioners) with a good general scientific education, a strong public health orientation, a well-developed social conscience and very broad clinical abilities.

In terms of the earlier discussion this reflects a well-developed community emphasis and this is evident in several aspects of the curriculum. Four afternoons per week of the first year are spent in inter-disciplinary workshops involving medical students, nurses and technicians studying 'Man – his environment', a programme designed to introduce the public health sciences. The fourth year involves some teaching of community health and this is followed in the fifth year by a community health assignment involving one-sixth of the class in villages remote from the medical school. The students work inter-professionally with health officers responsible for the health centres where the students are based.

Team training is fundamental to the Yaounde philosophy. The community health assignment is fundamental to this and has played a key role in adapting students to their leadership roles within health teams. In addition to this overtly community-based work there is a heavy emphasis on student research projects which are designed to develop research skills which will be of value in future careers.

AGA KHAN UNIVERSITY, KARACHI, PAKISTAN

This is a later example in a different country and in a recently established private university (Bryant *et al.* 1993). The system is different in that it is concerned with both the development of health care systems and with the education appropriate to their operation. Health care systems have been established in various rural and urban locations, some university-led, some government-led and others mixed in character. This allows for the interventions to be evaluated comparatively, but also creates a context in which the medical school or public health department is engaged with health care system development, making the integration of education and practice absolute in a way that is otherwise very difficult. Experience suggests that the interventions are producing health gains especially in the crucial area of child mortality.

On the teaching front there is a heavy emphasis on postgraduate development, but also a substantial segment of undergraduate medical and nursing degrees are occupied with public health concerns. Community health as it might be understood in a more developed context is less significant. From the perspective of long-established Western medical schools it is important to note that staff here have been recruited and trained into this approach rather than being converted from an established approach and thus avoid some of the defensive reactions towards curriculum change.

VELLORE, INDIA

As with most initiatives evaluation is seldom available, but this example does describe a fairly advanced approach to community-oriented education (Joseph and Abraham 1993). The approach features in years 1, 3, 4 and 5 of the course, with increasing autonomy being accorded to the student learner, and with a cumulative experience of the inter-sectoral and non-medical issues which are relevant to the community-based approach. The course also recognises the formal need for a multi-disciplinary approach, and the significance of cultural diversity as a part of community-based practice and education, issues which are equally important in most urban situations in developed countries. Once again, research is formally part of the curriculum as are management and planning in relation to health care.

XIAN MEDICAL UNIVERSITY, SHAANXI PROVINCE, CHINA

Discussion of this course suggests that its prime purpose, as with some of the examples in the United States, is to secure more doctors to work in rural areas (Umland *et al.* 1992). Unlike the other courses it does not appear to involve a particular community-oriented emphasis but is rather more about developing conventional practice in rural areas though it is also claimed that the course involves a heavy emphasis on preventive practice.

COMMUNITY-BASED EDUCATION

The earlier chapters have given some indication of the complex issues which the development of more community-oriented health care raise, and of the difficulties in defining precisely what that means. Equally they have made clear the problems in designing professional medical education to serve such developments and at the same time prepare for continuing professional development throughout long careers in what seems likely to be a volatile environment. The result has been a number of connected, but independent, educational developments. Some involve innovations in specific medical schools inspired by individuals, while others reflect a more general effort to innovate much more broadly, or at least to diffuse successful innovations more widely into reform of medical education on a national scale. These initiatives include explicit community-based education aimed at improved recruitment into that sector, or at producing doctors more competent to handle the roles involved in developing community-based medicine.

Alongside these emphases, and making analysis much more complicated, are other educational developments partly associated with that new emphasis and partly with the longer-term professional needs of all doctors. These developments include problem-based learning, self-directed learning, computer-assisted learning and other techniques designed to equip doctors for lifelong learning. Both of these patterns of development pose considerable challenges to the established way of doing things, and their own inter-connections are themselves complicated. Even where the reforms are aimed directly at supporting community-based medicine, they face problems of interpretation. The terms used have quite diverse meanings ranging from community-based learning which involves little more than using sites for learning in the community, to community education which carries much wider connotations. Where they aim to use new methods of teaching and learning, sometimes across the range of community-based education, then understanding what is happening is made much more difficult. It is therefore important to be clear about what is, and what is not, meant when community-based education is talked about in medicine and to clarify the distinction between that and the new learning methods also being introduced.

Before seeking to clarify this picture of change it is worth recognising the impact change may have on the traditional models of education which are being criticised. Two arguments were raised in defence of those models. One was that they were essential to meeting the need for competent doctors to work in the acute hospital sector. The other was that the more general nature of community-based practice meant that hospital-based learning was coincidentally adequate preparation for that role, though many in primary care would dispute that claim. Reform ideas which raise the possibility of a shift from hospital to community cause those within hospital-based specialities to question whether the reverse is also true and whether community-based learning can provide the experience appropriate to subsequent hospital working, often creating defensive reactions to many proposed changes. This debate raises basic questions about the nature of medical practice in both settings and the degree of difference in their approach. The answers should ideally be settled before decisions are taken about the overall character of any reformed professional education and about the timing and character of specialist preparation for each role. In some sense all medicine is practised in the community, even hospitals function in communities of some sort, and health care is certainly intended to be for the benefit of the community. The character of the medical facilities in which it is practised may differ by sector, and so may features of particular specialties, but the need for shared understanding across the whole of medicine is being more widely accepted.

Given the range of initiatives being canvassed and adopted in medical education, one of the obvious confusions is the failure to clarify the distinction between the *location* of educational and training activity, the *methods* being adopted in teaching and learning, and the intellectual and practical *content* being dealt with at different stages and locations in the process. It may be that clarification of this distinction will greatly assist our discussion of community-based education and establish more clearly the relationships among the many developments being tried.

The confusion is not new and has been the object of discussion arising in particular from an examination of a number of early examples of medical schools experimenting with curriculum change. In this case the concern was with the relationship between problem-based learning, an increasingly popular method of teaching, but one which builds on a view about the character of medical practice, and community-oriented education, which is about both location and substance. Richards and Fulop examined 10 examples of medical schools where both aspects were seen as being established and were able to isolate two non-overlapping groups. In five the orientation of the experimental curriculum was community-based while in the other five it involved problem-based learning (Richards and Fulop 1987). In commenting on this, Glick argues persuasively against those who think that the two are inextricably intertwined, suggesting that the community, rather than being an essential location for problem-based learning, may not even be the best location (Glick 1991).

Given such confusion, it may be worth examining some of the early innovations in the medical curriculum to see if they provide some clarification of the concepts involved and the main orientations of the innovators.

UNIVERSITY OF LINKÖPING, SWEDEN

An early example of curriculum reform in Europe was introduced at the University of Linköping in Sweden in 1986. As with so much reform in this area the motivation involved a number of issues related to traditional education. The prime emphases appear to have been adoption of the McMaster model of problem-based learning to take advantage of the benefits perceived to flow from that adult-learning model and thereby facilitate the involvement of six health care professions in an extensive shared learning (Areskog 1992). In addition to this, the course is regarded as 'more community-oriented than at other medical faculties in Sweden' (ibid.). The basis of this claim lies in the organisation of a considerable input from teacher/facilitators who are general practitioners and extended student experience in general practice settings and a course on Man–society which takes place in the first semester (Foldevi *et al.* 1994).

This combination of factors and approaches raises questions about the precise orientation involved, but comment by those involved suggests that it comes closer to replicating hospital experiences in a community setting rather than involving any wider conception of community in the approach. A clue to the approach lies in the expressed view that 'Primary care is a vital part of modern medicine, and problem-based learning/community-oriented medical education in general practice is the natural form of education for primary care' which seems to confuse two areas of focus and suggests a narrow view of primary care (Foldevi 1996). This means that

> During the first six terms the students assist at one of the health care centres around Ostergotland county within about 50 km from Linköping for half a day every week in order to get to know the primary health care setting, and to receive training in communicating with and in examining the patients.
>
> (Areskog 1992, pp.2–3)

It is evident that the community experience here is seen as essentially involving medicine in the community, with the individual patient as a prime focus, but echoing Iliffe in identifying 'general practice as a prime site for teaching all medicine, not just general practice' (Iliffe 1992). This is a perfectly laudable view but reflects a more limited conception of community-based learning than would, for example, be normal in those developing countries which have adopted this approach, some of which were considered earlier.

This is entirely consistent with the view that sees general practice as a context in which 'problem-solving' is the dominant mode of working and which therefore lends itself to the introduction of problem-based learning into the undergraduate curriculum. This approach to the use of the community is confirmed in Foldevi's later evaluations of the community aspect of the process, the clerkship in the community, which reflects very strongly the discussions about general practice education in the United Kingdom (Foldevi 1996). This evaluation also puts great emphasis on role modelling as a key aspect of this experience, but of course in any more radical orientation to medical education this should involve a much more careful selection of tutors, exposure to several role models, and a search perhaps for examples of more innovatory practice.

UK INNOVATIONS: KINGS COLLEGE AND CAMBRIDGE UNIVERSITY MEDICAL SCHOOLS

Kings College Medical School is one of the few innovative programmes which has looked at moving clinical teaching into the community. The ultimate aim is to create a community-based teaching hospital (an interesting conception itself), but at present students join an 8-week firm as part of their first year rotation. During this time students spend six sessions a week in the care of the community practice (with 1–2 students per practice) and two in complementary hospital sessions. In addition, students are also taken into casualty where they experience a variety of unsorted admissions.

The teaching and learning strategies adopted involve planned encounters between the students and patients either in the surgery, or at the patient's home, along with skills workshops where they explore such areas as learning methods and resources, case presentation methods, communication skills, clinical decision-making skills, planning patient management and evaluating clinical research. At the end of the 8 weeks students present a case study concerning an individually selected encounter, to both their peers and tutors. It is important to note that the general practitioner tutors follow a uniform systems-based teaching format organised in a similar manner to the hospital-based firms (McCrorie *et al.* 1993.)

The Cambridge University School of Clinical Medicine has pioneered a clinical course which will teach 50 per cent of the clinical skills/medical practice within a general practice setting. Although still in the experimental stage, this course appears successfully to address the problems associated with dwindling clinical material (patient numbers) in the hospital setting; providing protected teacher time and an opportunity for first-hand experience of the psycho-social effects of clinical medicine on the community.

Through the use of small group, one-to-one or peer group teaching involving direct observational study students are trained in the basics of clinical medicine and practice. Particular attention is given to the observation of systematic examination and the development of clinical problem-solving skills, as opposed to concentrating on purely physical signs. A substantial amount of the teaching is carried out by hospital specialists in conjunction with the treatment of practice patients, thus offering opportunities to follow practice patients to hospital out-patient and specialty departments, into wards and operating theatres. The emphasis therefore is on providing *integrated* clinical training rather than entirely replacing hospital-based training. After undertaking the conventional clinical introductory course students enter the new 'school' for training, returning briefly during the first clinical year to participate in the pathology course (McCrorie *et al.* 1993).

UNIVERSITY OF NEW MEXICO

In the United States the stimulus behind some more recent changes in the curriculum has been a concern with the limited numbers of doctors being recruited into family practice or primary care. This is explicit in the developments at the University of New Mexico which like the Swedish example emphasise self-directed, lifelong learning, but also seek 'to attract students to careers in primary care in rural and other underserved areas' (Kaufman *et al.* 1989, p.285). Once again the emphasis is like that in Sweden with community-oriented learning being seen as complementary to, rather than different from, hospital-oriented learning, and being more about a decision to 'expose students to the actual settings in which most will ultimately care for patients' (ibid.).

Community-based experience is built into the programme from the outset with a 4-month period off-campus forming the second part of the first year. Here the emphasis on individual practice in a community setting, with a tutor as role model and working in real clinics is very evident but in addition students will work on a community health project. These projects reflect a wider concept of community and the community setting is reported as stimulating an interest 'in issues such as occupational health, child abuse, and the effect of poverty on access to health care' (ibid., p.288), all of which suggest a widening of orientation reflecting a different aspect of the community setting.

Very properly this experiment in early medical education reform was extended to tackle the wider issues involved in a community orientation. Kaufman and his colleagues acknowledge that 'the focus has been on how students learn and on career choice with little emphasis on prevention of illness or on the health of the community as a whole.' (ibid., p.292). As with the example of Linköping, there is here a tendency to see problem-based learning as the key development, and the community as the best setting in which that may be developed.

MICHIGAN STATE UNIVERSITY

Here the curriculum includes a course on Primary Care Management for third-year students which initially looks like the approach being adopted in the British cases already discussed. In this case, however, the experience of working with community-based physicians is reinforced by a less usual component exposing the student to community agency contacts. This involves the students coming in contact with a wide range of agencies ranging from social services to support groups for specific illnesses. The key aspect of the contact is the requirement for students to report on an agency as part of the process of understanding 'how to explore and use community agencies to enhance their patients' care' (Potts 1994).

Evaluation of this clerkship indicated the high value which it offered in terms of enhancing student awareness of community agencies and increasing their likelihood of using such agencies in their treatment of patients. There was some discussion about the timing of the course, both within the medical school programme and in terms of the overall effort required of students. This reflected the felt need for students to have more experience for them to be able to make best use of the primary care clerkship. That may account for the fact that the learning appears to concentrate on particular agencies rather than addressing the more generic questions about community agencies and their value in relation to health and health care. More importantly from our point of view, despite this caveat, this is a programme which extends the idea of community relevance outside the formal health care institutions. It recognises the rich character of the community and the value that can have for the doctor in dealing with health care issues.

NORTH CAROLINA: MADISON COUNTY EXPERIMENT

This is a further example of a short elective in which the clinical experience of seeing patients with a physician mentor is extended into a more wide-ranging examination of the implications of the community setting. As described by Summerlin *et al.* (1993), half of each day is spent:

> collecting information about the community through existing data sources, community opinion polls, visits with home health nurses to individual patients' homes, visits to service agencies and community meetings, and attending meetings of the Community Advisory Board [the decision-making body for the Madison Community Health Program].

This exploration of the wider concept of community is further elaborated when students are invited to define and characterise the community through specific demographic, morbidity and mortality questions being asked about the area. Most specially 'Trainees have the opportunity to speak to political and other community leaders about their relationships to the community and its health care delivery system' (Summerlin *et al.* 1993). The outcome was that students and residents 'began to appreciate health as both a political and social community issue and a medical problem of individuals' (ibid.).

HARVARD MEDICAL SCHOOL

The New Pathways initiative at Harvard Medical School is different again. Its main emphasis is on innovatory learning methods like problem-based learning and intensive small group interaction, with only limited exposure to the community. At the same time the course does involve a wide range of subject matter which is highly relevant to a community orientation involving 'interweaving of material from the social and behavioural sciences, ethics, health promotion and disease prevention, and the humanities with teaching about clinical skills' (Moore *et al.* 1994). In terms of our typology, an extension of content with obvious community-based concerns, but no adequate matching experience within the community setting.

DISCUSSION

These examples serve to illustrate the limitations of the current innovations, but also confirm the confusion which exists about the community-based aspects of the different approaches being adopted. One thing which is clear is that community-based education is far removed from traditional medical education with its highly didactic teaching method, and narrowly defined substance related to the bio-medical model of medicine.

Several other things are also clear. Community-based education may be different, but like hospital-based teaching, it is not itself a method of teaching or of learning. A wide variety of learning methods are already in use in the context of existing provision and among the experiments in curriculum reform which have been established. In terms of method the existing style of general practice training is not very distinct from the experiential and apprenticeship-based aspects of medical school. The gaining of formally supervised experience is a central part of the process as is the engagement of one-to-one teaching and learning from that experience. Vocational trainees in the United Kingdom enjoy a half-day release course which takes the form of a facilitated group tutorial not unlike the system which prevails in medical school. Of course it is argued that the style of these experiences, and their content, are quite unlike medical school, but those are not issues of method but rather of the quality of the process and the nature of the content.

In much the same way, many of the experiments in the community involve project work and the preparation by students of formal written reports about their community experience. These sometimes involve teams of students working together, but again this is no different in principle from activity engaged within other settings. The issues may be different, the sources of information are different, and the orientation may inevitably be less scientific (certainly less bio-medical), but in terms of teaching methods this is quite a common educational experience.

There may be an argument which suggests that some methods are more easily engaged within the community setting. The character of practice, the nature of the setting and the significance of context make diagnosis and the establishment of cause more complicated than in much hospital care, with treatment equally complex as a result. These matters are not about teaching method, however, but derive from the location and from the factors which are relevant because of place.

Conventionally, in developed systems where there is a very elaborate institutional structure for care delivery, teaching in the community involves it taking place in one of those institutional settings. In these cases as was clear in the examples, the clinic, or health centre, becomes an alternative to the hospital, providing a flow of patients from whom the necessary skills for generic medical practice, and for community-based practice, may be learned. This is not to minimise the importance of the distinction between hospital and health centre practice. The educational possibilities in the different settings are quite different. The hospital provides the acute cases of established illness and focuses on narrow treatment of the condition. These factors dictate the scientific character of much of the work, perhaps explain the more didactic nature of much of the teaching, and the institutional setting inhibits the impact of the community context within which the hospital operates, but from which it is in some measure isolated. This is particularly the case with teaching hospitals with their wider catchments, more selective patient lists, and often their detailed location, all of which condition access and complicate the context. It is worth noting that this need not, and perhaps should not be the case. Speedier discharge, on the one hand, and the growth of emergency admissions, on the other, are two issues which bind the hospital much more closely into its geographical context. They are made much more complicated by the fact that they are often handled without the benefit of professional awareness of the community context which is relevant but which has been absent from professional training in the past.

Of course it is the case that the community can offer a much wider array of medical, and related non-medical, facilities in which education and training could take place. It remains the case, however, that these are not heavily used and where they are it is often not a working experience, marking their distinction from formal medical placements, but limiting the impact of such placements in an educational process where experiential learning and supervised practice loom so large. This focuses very clearly the question of aim and purpose in relation to community education, a matter to which we will return.

Aim and purpose focus the debate much more sharply and, if they are widened, provide a different justification for the community orientation discussed in relation to much curricular innovation. For many of the established examples of community-based education the aim and purpose are inherent in the activity itself. Primary care training is about preparing qualified doctors for work in a setting with which they are largely unfamiliar. Undergraduate attachments to general practice or family medicine are an approach intended to modify that degree of ignorance by providing some awareness of what such practice is like. Some of the specialty experience in the community provides an opportunity for intending hospital doctors to become aware of the context from which their patients will come, and to acquire a closer understanding of some of the issues which may influence health and disease.

The point about these experiences is that they continue to focus on the individual patient and the doctor's prime role in dealing with such patients. Of course the community experience raises wider questions than those which arise in a limited stay, acute episode of hospital care, but they remain a context for the individual case. Public health medicine is the most obvious context in which the wider concept of community becomes relevant. They are the doctors who deal with aggregates, with the more general issues of causation in terms of disease patterns within the community. They tend to be the doctors who deal with a wider range of institutions in their role in the promotion of health, the prevention of disease, and the handling of health-related issues. In short, community for the public health specialist is quite different from community conceived in relation to primary care or other areas of care in which a community orientation is being advocated.

It would seem from this discussion that community is a context in which a diverse substantive agenda might be pursued, but that a community orientation *per se* does not dictate that agenda. Many possibilities are embraced within what is called a community orientation. It then seems that the chosen agenda will be the instrument which dictates the specific locations in which learning will take place, and the methods which will be adopted to pursue that learning. There is no singular model of community-based learning. It means different things to different people, and in different settings.

It was clear in Chapter 2 that there is already a great deal of community-based health care and in consequence a number of developed models of community-oriented education in place preparing current professionals for a variety of non-hospital roles. The elaborate system of training for general practice in the United Kingdom has already been outlined, illustrating what might be called medical education in a specific community setting. In addition, there is the training currently available to intending public health specialists whose orientation is less to a specific community setting than to a range of issues which relate to community health. These are quite distinct models, engage quite different ideas about communities, and train professional staff in quite distinct areas of knowledge and skill deemed relevant for their main roles.

There are emerging examples of these principles being extended to doctors training within other specialisms where it is deemed relevant to have experience outside hospitals. Paediatrics looms large in this context, and there are some other cases which suggest that the different setting may throw up enough case experience to qualify specialists adequately, but also generate another agenda derived from the community which is relevant to the long-term career (Charney 1994).

It is worth spending a little time to clarify what this range of options involves and how best we might conceive of community education when it is applied to the basic generic education of medical students. This brings us immediately face to face with the issue of what knowledge, skills and attitudes it is felt are appropriate to establish in young medical students and how the community setting relates to those. Examination of much writing about community-based education currently reveals a clear tension between the community as a place where primary care is learned about and one in which the basics of generic medical practice are established. The former builds on the historical model which suggests two quite different orientations, but in which the community orientation has been under-valued. The idea that all doctors should develop awarenesses and skills within the community, whether they work in primary or in secondary care, assumes a novelty value in that traditional context.

4

Aims and purposes of
community-based education

The debate about community-based medical education reflects a number of divisions within medical education. First is the dominant concern, shared with other professions, with the initial stages of professional education. The community orientation has been decidedly lacking within the undergraduate medical curriculum in the past so that its introduction there implies a quite radical agenda for many of those involved. Second is the relatively weak position of the community-based specialisms within the medical hierarchy. The arguments for, and the practice of, community-based postgraduate education for those specialisms have been established for some years but have had little impact on the undergraduate curriculum during that time. Third is the relatively limited attention given to continuing medical education and the institutional problems of catering for professional needs in the highly pressured context of health care provision. Despite this it remains true that community-based practitioners, and indeed some hospital-based specialists who have developed community-based practice, engage their continuing professional education and development in the community. In short, there is already quite a lot of community-based education around in medicine, some of it concentrated in obvious community-based specialties, and much of it undertaken informally and outside the formal professional educational institutions.

These largely professional concerns are often difficult to resolve, but resolution is made more difficult by the fact that they are increasingly reinforced by external pressures for medicine to change. This is reflected in the range of motivations to be found among those currently seeking to promote community-based education within medical education generally and in the undergraduate curriculum in particular. These motivations range from concerns, inside and outside the profession, about the organisation of health care service delivery, in terms of quantity and quality, cost and equity, to concerns about the changing character of the services delivered and the needs of future doctors called upon to play new roles within this changing context. Such motivations have obvious implications for the undergraduate careers of medical students, but the situation also relates to the need to equip doctors with the skills and attitudes to cope with the career-long challenges in their personal and professional development. These different motives are closely inter-related, but it is important to clarify the distinctions if community-based education is to develop in ways which will satisfy future needs.

GENERAL AIMS

At the most pragmatic level the shortage of community-based doctors, in primary care and other specialties, is one important driving force for change. This is particularly evident in the United States which 'Among Western industrialized nations ... ranks last in providing primary health care services' (Herold *et al.* 1993) and which has undertaken a good deal of curriculum innovation to try to influence student choice of specialty. It has not been such an obvious issue elsewhere, though evidence has been appearing in the United Kingdom since the mid-1990s which suggests that there is now a problem there both in terms of the recruitment of new general practitioners and retention of those already in practice. Such problems also appeared in the 1960s and were met then by the GPs Charter and the development of a system of postgraduate training for general practice. Solutions are now seen as lying partly within initial professional education and so reform of the undergraduate curriculum is being seen as having an important contribution to make. Such changes concentrate on the narrow issues of doctor education, but wider issues about the organisation and staffing of primary care may also be relevant to the problem, and so to the solution, and they may require the undergraduate curriculum to be adapted in other more radical ways.

It is interesting to see that the profession sees greater experience of community-based practice during early training as being an encouragement to young doctors to opt for community-based careers despite the evidence of stress and disillusion among many current community practitioners. This optimism rests of course on assumptions about those who will teach within the community setting and the quality of the experience they can offer and the work which they demonstrate to medical students. The model of postgraduate vocational education is often induced as the basis for such arguments but there is evidence that the model does not always work well even at the postgraduate level, and that other issues are important to decisions about medical careers.

Such considerations are also relevant when other broad motivations for introducing community-based education are being considered. One set of these is concerned with the quality of current practice within the community and the aim of reform is to equip doctors better for undertaking such established roles. This addresses the argument often heard within general practice about the inappropriate nature of much current medical education for careers to be spent in the community. This may involve little more than providing much more direct student experience of the two community-based specialties, primary care and public health, though there would be much coincidental value from community experience in other specialties where community-based practice is developing. Charney, for example, points out the degree to which paediatrics in the United States involves practice from offices within the community, and, as we shall see, advocates community-based education in a primary care setting for doctors aiming at this specialty (Charney 1994).

In this formulation the aim of community-based education is to provide direct, supervised experience of the current specialty in the setting where it is normally practised. It involves an extension of the principles which underlie hospital-based medical education, though as we will see, the implications of work in the community setting extend the agenda in important ways. This approach is already evident in the postgraduate training of general practitioners in most developed countries where a period, usually a year, in a general practice is required. The character of the engagement is different in the case of public health, but the essence of the system is very much the same, as would also be the case where other specialties work in the community. The consultant moving out of hospital to offer sessions within a general practice, or from his or her own office, will surely have to engage with a wider range of issues in dealing with patients than was the case when they worked within secondary/tertiary care.

Such preparation is currently seen as a postgraduate option once doctors have achieved their basic qualification. Translation of the idea of providing such experience in the undergraduate curriculum and how it might need to be adapted and modified to serve the needs of medical students is the challenge facing curriculum reformers. For many within medicine, the proposed change of emphasis arises simply from the overwhelming dominance of hospital experience in current education, and the need to secure a balance between the sectors. This can lead to a view being taken of reform which sees the necessary community experience as being like the current hospital experience, with the community surgery substituting for the ward as the site of learning. This view tends to emphasise current practice and accepts the value of apprentice experience of such practice which lies at the core of the traditional medical model discussed earlier. As was suggested then, it is desirable that this should be well done if it is to form the core base of qualification to practice in the community. This in itself poses a challenge as there is no intrinsic reason to suppose that community-based teaching will necessarily be better in quality than hospital-based teaching which has been the object of much criticism. Recruitment and selection of teachers and their training will be central to the success of any changes introduced.

Such changes may have considerable benefit for the quality of current practice. What they may not do is prepare students for future practice which may differ widely from the current model. This raises a range of other considerations. Three aspects of the future merit consideration. First is the fact that the current community-based practice is not fixed, nor is it so narrowly focused as might appear from the patterns of existing professional training. Initial practice may be concerned with the ability to work in isolation, in an uncertain context and to diagnose, treat or refer with safety, but more mature practice demonstrates a widening of the role to embrace a range of other activity. This widening of role demands that consideration be given to the initial experience in the community if it is to equip the doctor adequately for the wider role, or it must provide the initial building blocks which enable the doctor to engage with the widening as it occurs. This is partly about individual capacity, but there is also a need for the system and the organisations involved to facilitate this process.

Second, there is the need to anticipate the changing context of health care in the community and the extent to which that will alter current practice. Some of this is already manifest in changes in the structure of the primary care system, the demands of managed care, and the significant changes within hospital care which are having effects in the community. The emergence of patterns of care provided by a range of professional staff working together raises a large number of issues for the nature of community-based medical practice which all have educational implications. Team-working with other professions and the issues of resource management in such a situation afford obvious examples. The audit and research demands generated by such changes and the pressure for evidence-based practice are obvious corollaries. The implications for community-based education where the aims address this longer-term future are challenging.

Third, and relevant to both the earlier themes, is the need to cater for the lifetime learning needs of the doctor in training. This is not inherently a question which derives from community-based education or practice, as it is an important issue for those practising in hospitals as well. It does mean that alongside the direct concern with those issues which arise because the education is community-based is an agenda about educational method and style which embraces this longer-term aim. One test of the value of community-based education may be its capacity to deliver such coincidental educational goals.

PARTICULAR AIMS

These broad aims for community-based education are not of course matched in practice, even in those medical schools who have been in the vanguard of curriculum change. In part this is accounted for by their very generality. There is a need to be more specific about educational reform and to provide some analytical basis for understanding existing changes and promoting future development. This is doubly important because community-based education carries no necessary implications for the nature and character of what occurs by way of teaching or of learning. Just as hospital-based education may be better or worse, so too may education in the community.

Even within the context of existing primary care provision the education and training involved vary widely, and whatever the rhetoric, the outcome tends ultimately to focus on quite a narrow range of priority goals. At the heart of much community-based education, for example, is the patient and the development of student capacity for dealing with individual patients. In essence this is the same for hospital or community practice. The difference lies in the factors which may be seen to be relevant in the community setting, and which are less likely to be seen within the hospital, though not necessarily so. In essence the issue is what factors the community setting places on the agenda, or in most cases, places on the potential agenda, which are likely to be excluded within the hospital context by the nature of the treatment being offered.

Most obviously the community involves a potential broadening of perspective. In terms of the treatment of individual patients this means seeing them within the context of their family and in relation to their wider position in the community. Awareness of this contextual information, and the case management which takes it into account, lie at the basis of what is regarded as good quality community-based care. This is in sharp contrast to the hospital where the focus is narrowed to concentrate on the diagnosed condition and where the shortening of hospital treatment times is reinforcing that narrowing of concern. In addition, the wider community context itself has relevance for community-based practice. Health and health care go beyond the treatment of individual cases as and when they occur. Populations manifest varied health profiles giving rise to community-based interventions to prevent illness, educate about health, and treat pro-actively rather than re-actively. This concern for 'population medicine' may be extended into 'public health' medicine where the agenda widens significantly to embrace non-health sectors and their significance for health. Community-based learning is appropriate for any or all of these extended orientations.

The diverse motivations for introducing more community-based learning into medical education with these divergent aims and objectives raise equally varied possibilities in terms of what might be included within the revised curriculum. On the one hand, they involve students in an extended version of the traditional clinical curriculum, but at the other extreme involve them in dealing with quite different domains of knowledge from those traditionally taught.

In that context the broad, generalised aims do not help much in the analytic sense as both may be served in a wide variety of ways, in a wide variety of settings, and using a wide range of techniques for learning and teaching. This gives added significance to discussion about aims and objectives, forcing much more rigorous debate about the nature of community-based practice and the knowledge, skills and attitudes which might best serve those involved.

In seeking to bring greater clarity to the debate a number of distinctions may be made. One common distinction is between those issues which are relevant to the professional development of medical students, and those which are relevant to their personal development. Both are relevant to community-based practice, but personal development is often seen as having particular relevance to the patient–doctor relationship advocated in general practice. Looking at the professional aspects there are a number of aspects involved.

First, and most obvious, is the learning of primary care practice, an objective which may easily lead to the uncritical adoption of ideas and approaches to both practice and education which are to be found in current postgraduate training and education. The danger with any such simple adoption is that the number of students involved in undergraduate education is much larger, the students are much less mature than their postgraduate counterparts and perhaps more importantly, the assumption that current primary care practice is both satisfactory and provides a sound learning environment for those who will practise in the future may be misplaced. The significance of these issues is increased by the prevalence of the one-to-one, apprentice model of postgraduate education, and the heavy emphasis on experiential learning in that current mode. A more rigorous view of the relevance of this model, and of ways in which it might be modified, may be achieved if the different aspects of primary care are examined more closely. Charney elaborates some of these features in considering community-based education for paediatricians and distinguishes three areas of learning in what he characterises as 'patient centred, office centred and physician centred' activities (Charney 1994). His more detailed outline of particular elements within each of these areas is shown in Table 4.1.

It should be remembered that Charney is concerned with the training of specialist paediatricians to work in the community so that the emphasis may differ from that of the generalist community physician. That may help to explain the individualised nature of the examples outlined under each heading although many within generalist community practice would echo the same emphasis. The importance of Table 4.1 is that it highlights the importance of all three aspects of community practice as part of the training package. Taken together, they provide a broad outline of community-based practice but they begin to hint at an extension of the traditional role in various ways. Such extensions would be more evident if the example related directly to generalist community practice.

In terms of patient-centred objectives the continuity of primary care is very evident, together with an awareness of the need for shared care in providing a comprehensive range of services for chronically ill patients in the community. The care of low severity/high frequency conditions is different, though again, management over time is likely to focus attention on wider questions of patient education and awareness. One aspect of such concerns is recognised in the emphasis placed on health promotion and disease prevention which are acknowledged as significant aspects of community-based care which arise more obviously where care is continuous and the patient context well understood.

Communication skills underpin all of these activities in so far as they involve work with individual patients. It is of note that Charney gives little hint of any more collective approaches to these issues, whether of broad local populations or of the whole patient population, a comment which would apply as much to primary care as to community paediatrics. In this formulation community-based training is about learning to deal with individual patients, albeit in a different way from much traditional practice, but does not reflect the wider orientations discussed earlier, despite

Table 4.1 *What can be learned in community primary practice settings*

Patient-centered objectives	Health promotion/disease prevention
	Care of low-severity/high-frequency conditions
	Care of chronic disease (shared care)
	Care of patients over time (when to consult, refer)
Office-centered objectives	Variety of practice models (solo, group, urban, rural)
	Use of office records
	Use of parent/patient education materials
	Telephone management
Physician-centered objectives	Physicians' role in community (schools, day-care facilities, parent groups)
	Physicians' role in community hospital
	'Life and times' of practitioner

Source: Charney (1994, p.667)

clear recognition elsewhere that the community setting ideally involves a much wider perspective.

Turning to office-centred objectives, the broader population perspective does not appear here either, but there is more of a sense of the practice setting being an important aspect of the practitioner's work. This is evident in the consideration given to practice location, and the size of the practice team, and to some formal issues of management and of record keeping. Though not spelt out, such factors implicitly raise questions about the nature of the staff involved in practice and how issues of teamwork are best engaged. In this formulation these issues are presented as office-based, but they do also raise issues about professional practice and the character of health care, or they do in teams where several professions are involved, as is becoming more common in primary care. These issues look more like physician-centred ones in this formulation though they do not arise formally in that context. Such matters certainly highlight the importance of the practice setting, though the fact that this is community-based is not itself considered formally.

The physician-centred objectives revert to the narrower perspective and are concerned with what community-based paediatricians, and more generally family physicians, currently do. In a sense these overlap with the patient-centred objectives, but more critically they reflect a static model of primary care and contrast somewhat with the more developmental office-centred objectives. It is certainly the case with current vocational training for general practice that the emphasis lies heavily within the mix of patient and physician-centred objectives, with most office-centred learning being left until after formal qualification. The prioritising of such features tells us a great deal about community paediatrics, and by extension about perceptions of much primary care, summed up in the phrases which are often used about 'safe doctors' and 'preparation for independent practice' during vocational training for general practice. In many ways the office-based objectives refer to inter-dependent practice, or what might currently be termed multi- or inter-professional practice. Unless those office-based perspectives are emphasised, community-based education on this model becomes little more than a balancing of training experience in favour of the general practice surgery as opposed to the hospital clinic or ward.

This conception is extended if one takes the second feature of the professional side of the equation which involves a different conception of medicine compared with that applied in hospital. From this perspective, the different setting and the different nature of the conditions which are confronted there focus attention onto a wider bio-psycho-social model of medicine (Engel 1977). This involves the student in extending the scope of patient consultation beyond the narrower hospital focus to retain the biological factors, but also to recognise their inter-connection with psychological and social factors which derive from the patient's family and community position. This is particularly significant where the care of the particular patient will continue over time, unlike the acute hospital experience with its shorter-term provision of health care. This widened perception of both cause and treatment of disease demands different diagnostic tools, and certainly different approaches to treatment.

The effect of this widening goes further. The hospital doctor is oriented to disease, and in the main sees only those patients who have been screened and referred as probably suffering from some disease which needs treatment of a more complex kind. In contrast, the open direct accessibility of community practice means that a wide range of conditions are seen, some patients are well although the service may be medicalised (childbirth) and many have only minor conditions which demand modest or limited treatment. It is this 'normal' distribution of patients which makes the community experience so different from hospital, but which also adds a further dimension to community practice. The normal distribution does nothing to limit the uncertainty associated with particular cases. The aggregate distribution of cases clearly involves many who are well or only mildly indisposed but the skill of community practice is to deal with those minor conditions but also to detect the rarer cases where the diagnosis is more serious and merits a referral. This is made more complicated by the fact that ill health and its causes extend widely, taking diagnosis and treatment outside the realm of purely medical care to include a wide range of other knowledge and referrals consistent with the holistic view taken of the patient within the community setting.

Some authors have extended this wider conception of the medical role even further to embrace the idea of comprehensive care which takes in other aspects of the community experience. Iliffe and Zwi have suggested that the medical graduate should be able to incorporate a 'social, psychological and anthropological understanding of health and disease' into their diagnosis and treatment, the anthropological bringing a key element of community understanding into consideration (Iliffe and Zwi 1994). They go further to argue that the doctor who is to work in the community must also understand how health services respond to the needs of the population if they are to operate sensitively in referring patients. This conception may be extended beyond health services into many other areas if the full richness of community need and service opportunity are to be engaged.

These widening perspectives involve doctors moving from a focus on the individual patient to take a population-based view of their role, reflecting some of the earlier discussion about office-based objectives and about prevention and patient education or participation. This begins to move the discussion towards the other area of professional practice which lies firmly within the community orientation, that of the public health doctor. Some of the complexity of the earlier discussion arises in part from the fact that there are several medical roles played in the community which are quite rigidly demarcated at the present time despite recognition that such rigid divisions do not reflect the way communities are organised and operate. In much the same way as was argued for primary care, public health also covers a wide range of possible action. On the one hand, it involves an emphasis on prevention, on health promotion and education, but also includes a wider concern with the impact on people's health of factors which fall outside the concerns of conventional health care. This range is reflected in their concern with the maintenance of health in the wider population rather than with individual patients (Kark and Kark 1983). This focus on the 'entire community' compares sharply with concern for the individual patient, or even with the list of registered patients which tends to characterise primary care (Todd 1992). It focuses attention on the need to understand those people who 'do not regularly find their way into the general practitioner's consulting room' (Greenlick 1992), for example those with AIDS, alcohol and drug misusers, and some ethnic minorities excluded from conventional care programmes for one reason or another.

These extensions of concern involve a parallel extension of the knowledge base needed for such practice, involving a range of new disciplines and the acquisition of new skills which are needed for wider population-based, or public health, practice. For example, it is common to see community-based learning as an opportunity to develop better and more effective communication skills, but this is usually seen as only relevant to the consultation. The point about community-based practice is that it involves a much wider interaction with other professions and other agencies and the use of new channels for communication. It also involves different types of message, certainly if there is to be a transition to more population-based practice. These wider considerations raise an important agenda for medical education and training, but it is one which is often crowded out by the concentration on using the community setting as a venue for learning basic clinical skills which are either not taught, or are not well taught, in hospital settings. The community setting is one place where this might be done, but experience with clinical skills laboratories suggests that this may be done in many settings and is not dependent on taking place in the community physician's surgery.

These professional objectives are matched by a range of personal development objectives which may be considered independently. As they are treated in the current literature these involve a number of features, some of which fall at the boundary with professional skills. First is the need to develop appropriate orientations and attitudes among medical students which will equip them for a long career in medicine. It is argued that this will be fostered by a broad-ranging experience with a wide cross-section of patients and with a wide range of associated professional colleagues. There is little doubt that the community provides a context in which this is more likely to happen, and more importantly, where continuing relationships require more awareness in initial contacts with both groups of people. This is particularly the case in the context of more complex populations where multi-cultural issues can arise, especially in urban areas (Pereira Gray 1994 and GMC 1993).

Another personal development often discussed in the context of community-based education is the need to develop appropriate learning styles for a lifetime of practice. In the main this implies the development of self-directed learning capacities, and for some commentators these are best engaged within the community setting. There is little doubt that the setting would cater for such capacity building, but equally little doubt that such capacity could also be developed within the hospital setting. The emphases of the latter, as we have seen, tend towards models of medicine and of diagnostic analysis which may well depend less on these learning capacities and much more on directed learning of large volumes of material. It is equally the case that over a long hospital career there will be a need to deal with new developments and changing situations, all of which would benefit from self-directed learning skills. This like so much else in this context reflects the tendency to categorise hospital-based learning as though it has inherently to be like it has been in the past rather than as needing to be adapted to a different future. Positing the community as the place where relevant skills are learned could leave hospital-based medicine where it currently is, despite a need to cultivate better communication, more population awareness, and many other characteristics in that setting as well as in relation to community-based practice itself.

ARGUMENTS FOR COMMUNITY-BASED EDUCATION

A more defined set of subsidiary aims arise from the range of broad objectives discussed in the last section. They concern the subject base of a curriculum which would prepare doctors for the range of roles discussed. The question of what should be taught in medical school has a long pedigree, as was commented earlier, but the traditional debate has been largely conducted about the traditional core of bio-medical sciences. There have been periodic additions to the list of subjects taught, but the inability to agree about removing any existing subjects, or even to change the ways in which they are taught and assessed, has made it difficult to make significant changes. In part, the problem has been dealt with by leaving some areas to be taken up in specialist postgraduate study as is the case with epidemiology for public health or aspects of management for some members of varied specialties. This has been most marked in the community-oriented specialties which accounts in some measure for the current concern to change the undergraduate core more radically than has been possible in the past. The fragmentation inherent in the postgraduate model does little to enhance the working relationships between the different community specialties, nor between them and the traditional hospital specialties, inhibiting relationships which are seen as increasingly important. This becomes even more significant in relation to the increasing discussion about community-based practice in the future. This is beginning to hint at a model of future community-based practice which moves beyond the current efforts at reform designed to meet immediate shortcomings. This debate is instructive in clarifying the wider perspective in which community-based education needs to be set.

One variant of that debate is taking place within the context of general practice within the United Kingdom. Several commentators (Irvine 1993; Boaden 1997) have observed the need to incorporate a much wider professional base in the vocational training of doctors and the most recent government statements about primary care reinforce that need (Secretary of State for Health 1997). This reflects recognition of the fact that the community-based career may start out dominated by the provision of individual patient care, but that it develops in many directions as experience, personal preferences and the changing context of practice shape professional development. Many of the options discussed remain close to conventional practice, but others move the debate from a concern with Charney's patient and professional concerns towards the wider concerns with the practice and the primary health care team. All are features which benefit greatly from community-based experience for their fullest exploration, though it is worth remarking that some, like team-work, are equally central to much hospital care, where inter-professional development is every bit as relevant as it is in the community. What most such discussions do not do is embrace the wider subject content inherent in the extended model of primary care being considered as one option here.

This is taken up by some commentators who look forward to practice in the twenty-first century in a more general way. In an analysis based on the need for quite different orientations in the education of doctors for practice in that century, Greenlick elaborates some of the characteristics which he sees as inherent in a more community-oriented practice and consequently in education for such practice. These do not remove the central concern with offering the best available treatment to patients, but are seen as important additions to that core continuing activity. They include the following:

- an economic or resource allocation component;
- a component focusing on the epidemiological aspects of new practice;

- a component focusing on members of the population who do not regularly find their way into the physician's office or whose needs are not attended to within the normal context.

(Greenlick 1992, p.182)

Such elements occur in many commentaries on future educational needs and are beginning to appear in some medical school curricula. For example, Greenlick cites with approval the developments at Harvard Medical School which involve students in acquiring a range of competencies which he and they deem essential to the future practice of medicine, namely:

- the ability to manage information;
- the ability to manage care resources;
- the ability to work as part of a team;
- the ability to integrate guidelines and clinical judgement and to 'manage to outcomes'.

(ibid.)

Superficially these may appear quite like some more traditional goals, but their significance within the emerging ideas about community-based practice is potentially very radical.

Such concerns find an echo in the subject content of curricula where the demands of community-based practice are being considered though in these formal terms the list can often look quite formidable. Hiatt and Goldman (1994) raise another significant aspect of such developments in their discussion of what they call the 'evaluative medical sciences' which they regard as being inadequately taught. This highlights a key dilemma in the extension of the professional curriculum into domains of subject matter which essentially fall within other disciplines and so other professions. This may account for their list of things which are badly taught in medical school which features statistics, epidemiology, decision analysis, cost-effectiveness analysis, economics and computer sciences. It may seem more surprising that the list also includes health services research and ethics which might appropriately be seen as falling more clearly within the traditional medical education agenda.

This brief discussion of some of the extended possibilities related to community-based education highlights the fact that delivery of such education will require more radical decision-making than is normal within professional education. It suggests that reform engaged within the profession, and within the traditional medical schools, may well fall short of what is needed to make the radical changes which health care reform suggests are necessary. This may become clearer in the next chapter when the settings for such extended education are considered.

5

Settings for community-based learning

It is clear from the discussion of aims and objectives in the last chapter that community-based education is a complex matter. Despite its obvious wide-ranging potential, as we shall see, much current innovation is driven by relatively modest objectives and arises within the well-established professional framework which adopts a relatively narrow primary care model of community-based health care. This rather conservative approach no doubt reflects the difficulties involved in establishing change, both within the institutions of medical education and across the structure of health care with their long-established patterns of professional dominance and relatively poor inter-agency and inter-professional cooperation. The significance of these aspects of current practice is that they are much more central to community-oriented health care, hence the current drive towards reform. This is reflected very well in consideration of the settings within which community-based education does, and in the future might, take place. This chapter considers the range of community settings in which community-based education is currently undertaken, and more importantly, the much wider range of potential venues available if it is to address the extended set of aims and objectives outlined earlier.

As we saw earlier, one strong argument advanced in favour of community-based education sees its main purpose as being to complement and balance the existing emphasis on hospital-based experience. This perspective seems to involve finding community settings for education which may be treated in a way analogous to that in which hospital settings are used. This is precisely the model which applies in relation to postgraduate training for primary care now, for example, in the case of general practice in the United Kingdom. Undergraduate education is in the main failing to provide adequate opportunities for students to see, and experience, primary care in the community. Vocational training compensates for that by providing supervised experience within the confines of a surgery located in the community. It is worth noting that the availability of surgery space for the vocational trainee is one of the requirements placed on training practices. Given this emphasis many characteristics of the community-based consultation are not essentially different from those which apply in a hospital, although those working in general practice argue that the nature of the interaction with patients is entirely different. The significance of the consultation taking place 'in the community' they argue, lies not in the location but in the character of the interactions which take place. This depends, of course, on the degree to which patients bring and are encouraged to bring, or doctors seek out, the relevance of the community setting for diagnosis and treatment. In some cases, house calls may bring out the importance of contextual factors but they form only a limited part of practice, and recent changes in practice in the United Kingdom have meant that many such calls are now not undertaken by the patient's regular doctor. This begins to undermine arguments about continuity of care which have been used to sustain the importance of community-based practice, and experience in some more hospital-based specialties such as psychiatry or geriatrics raises similar concerns as community factors clearly have a bearing on patient treatment. More generally, the tendency for earlier discharge of patients from hospital care is making such matters increasingly important within all hospital specialties. This blurring of sector boundaries makes community experience more widely relevant, but the nature of the appropriate experience then needs more careful consideration. It does mean that confinement to the community surgery is not an appropriate substitute, or complement, to confinement on the hospital ward as a basis for training.

Even in relation to the narrowly defined current medical role in primary care, this emphasis on patient contact within the surgery has limiting effects, particularly in relation to developing skills in those central aspects of primary care such as continuity and comprehensiveness (Starfield 1992). These are the areas where current care patterns widen to involve other doctors, other health care professionals and some who do not fall within the conventional areas of health care. In relation to the wider aims of community-based education discussed in the last chapter, it is even more limited. Two conceptions of community may be distinguished at this point. One conceives of community in terms of the organisations and agencies which operate there with the geography of particular communities often being defined by the arbitrary choice of institutional boundaries. The problems of overlap and the confusion of responsibility for patients in some areas have often caused problems. The other approach conceives community in relation to the perceptions of residents, defining community by some sense of shared identity and focus, giving rise to quite different issues than those which arise in the first case. There is much evidence that for many people their sense of identification is with a very small 'community' often not consistent with the scale necessary for the provision of services for those living in that small area.

Taking the agency perspective and seeking to widen the range of settings within which community-based learning might be based, Figure 5.1 outlines the characteristics of location which may be relevant in light of earlier discussion. Six dimensions

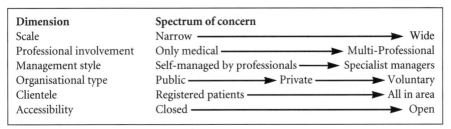

Dimension	Spectrum of concern
Scale	Narrow ———————————————➤ Wide
Professional involvement	Only medical ———————————➤ Multi-Professional
Management style	Self-managed by professionals ——➤ Specialist managers
Organisational type	Public ——————➤ Private ————➤ Voluntary
Clientele	Registered patients ———————➤ All in area
Accessibility	Closed ————————————————➤ Open

Figure 5.1 *Key dimensions and spectrum of concern involved in a choice of community settings.*

are distinguished and together might be seen as providing a template from which to match the setting with the aims and objectives of any community-based experience. One dimension is the professional orientation of the setting. This may range from the exclusively medical, through settings where other professions are working, or where non-professionals are involved, to those where multi-professional activity is the core of established practice. A second concerns the scale at which the organisation is established which might range from the regional base of a large hospital, through agencies working at the more local scale of a city, or of a large area, to the smaller sub-local level where agencies serve quite small numbers of people, not always as in general practice, living in a geographically exclusive area. A third dimension involves the management style of the organisation. Once again the range is diverse with some organisations managed by the professional staff while others are managed by 'professional managers', some are managed by politicians, others by lay management committees. A fourth dimension relates to the type of organisation involved which may be characterised in various ways. The significance is apparent, however, in the simple range from public sector to the private sector, with the voluntary organisation often conceived as lying somewhere in between. These categories themselves are not singular and have, if anything become more diverse, with complicated funding systems and public–private partnerships blurring some of the clear traditional distinctions. Finally, there are issues about the clientele of organisations, whether they cater for all, or only some of the relevant population, and whether access to the agency is open and determined by the client, or closed and the determined by gatekeepers within or outside the organisation itself.

The implications of these dimensions will be clearer if we consider some real examples of community settings looking at the different dimensions.

SCALE

It is helpful to remember the extent to which institutions vary along all the six dimensions being considered here with scale providing perhaps the most obvious example. The hospital–general practice dichotomy could not be more acute. The district general hospital may serve a 'community' of 300 000 people, a figure which may be appropriate to support its acute, specialist functions, but which has important implications in relation, for example, to accident and emergency services with their more open access to the whole population served. Even the smaller, cottage, or community hospital may serve a quite extended community, given the limited numbers of such hospitals and the perceived quality of the services which they can offer. In contrast the typical general practice may have 8–10 000 patients, but they will not constitute a community in any clear geographical sense except in the more remote rural setting. In inner cities the complexity of patient registration patterns and the greater prevalence of single-handed practitioners means that quite small communities are often served by a large number of practices. The implications for those working in the hospital setting create an obvious complexity in their agency relationships, but for those in the community these same features can be highly problematic. Certainly they can lend a competitive edge to access to hospital care, and they have an immediate effect on any more developed role in relation to population-based practice which requires extensive inter-practice cooperation or coordination for its achievement.

There is a need to be clear about these variations of scale, and the degree to which they overlap and inter-relate in seeking to find appropriate attachments for trainees whose professional practice when qualified will involve an understanding of the realities of popular use of health services. Effort will be needed so that professionals in training see examples of the range of orgnisations. It will also be necessary to structure such experience in ways which highlight the elements of organisation which are being examined and to provide real opportunities to assess their impact on professional practice.

PROFESSIONAL STAFFING

The staffing profile of agencies is in part related to the scale of operation just considered, but is more often a function of the historical evolution of national agency systems and the character of the professions involved. The model of the profession discussed earlier made great play of the need to possess characteristics which distinguish particular professional practitioners from others working in the area, basing that distinction on clearly defined knowledge, skills and training. An associated feature of the ideal–typical model of the professional is the continuation of that exclusivity into their practice. This is associated with practice organised around single professionals, or more latterly with groups drawn from the same profession, though often working as individuals within the group. The independent general practitioner, or dentist, or indeed solicitor or barrister, fits this model very well, and practice is organised around the chambers or the partnership with the professionals controlling their own activity.

These traditional professions have of course been joined by a wide range of others, or by a number of 'quasi-professions' often seeking to achieve what they regard as full professional status. More importantly for our discussion, many of these occupational groups have emerged with the development of public services associated with health care and related areas of social welfare. This combination of circumstances has led to a close correspondence between the structure of agencies and the development and exclusivity of professional roles. This led to the continued defence of independent practitioner status for general practitioners after 1948 in the United Kingdom and a range of separate organisations concerned with providing different community-based services. One consequence has been patterns of relatively isolated professional practice developing, defended as being necessary by the professions because of their wish to maintain professional autonomy. This has given rise to fragmentation of services in the past and has resulted in major failures of communication and great difficulties for some patients in being treated by a wide array of staff often with little effective coordination of their inputs. Such claims in light of such experience sit uncomfortably with current discussion about community-based care and inevitably mean that community-based education in the late 1990s will have to involve contact with, and experience of a large number of agencies if inter-professional practice is to develop.

More recently there has been some movement towards multi-professional work within the community and there are now more agencies where that can be found. These offer the advantage of opportunities for students to see professionals working within their own specialism, but in close association with other professions. Such working methods are an inherent feature of many of the proposed future models of community-based practice and their implications are obviously better understood if trainee professionals have experience in contexts where they already apply. Placements in community settings need to be arranged with this dimension of organisation clearly in mind, and also need to provide opportunities where joint working may be experienced.

MANAGEMENT STYLE

Similar arguments may be raised in relation to the question of management style within the varied agencies involved. The archetypal model of professional practice is the individual one of self-management where the concept of management in its general form is not relevant. The inhibitions inherent in such an isolated model of practice in today's complex society reflect the downside of such a model of professional autonomy and account for its increasing rarity within all the established professions. Single-handed practice in community medicine still remains, with the primary organisational task being the arrangement of appointments for the one practitioner. Even within small group practices that style continued until quite recently with a senior receptionist organising group appointments but a practice manager being relatively unusual. The professionals would 'manage' their own practice, individually, through a designated senior or executive partner, or as a partnership, dealing with any other managerial tasks necessary to their practice. This concept of self-management is being overtaken by a range of external demands being made on practices, concerned with accountability, resource use and extended team-work, and most particularly in relation to financial developments, which are together promoting the concept of general management within community-based medical practice.

The larger, and often more extended, variant of practice through a primary health care team calls for much more by way of management capacity, although it remains the case that much inter-professional work is managed by referral rather than by mutual decision and organised resource use. Increasingly, there is recognition of the role of a manager to deal with the issues which arise in such complex team settings, though as Huntington makes clear there is still a doubt as to 'whose business' it is to manage (Huntington 1995). This reflects the long-standing difficulty many professionals experience with the idea of their work being managed, and the limitations which they see management as placing on their professional autonomy.

The culture of practice is quite different in many of the other settings where community-based education might be experienced and where the professions involved are less developed in the formal sense. Most are subject to more conventional models of management, with clear hierarchies of responsibility and accountability, and a very clear division of labour. The educational importance of this distinction is that these features characterise many of the agencies with which community physicians need to work and it is the understanding of their different character and *modus operandi* which is so important. Such features may also come to characterise the working environments of community-based doctors in the future if some models of community-based care are adopted.

Other aspects of organisations are also important. It is striking within the hospital sector in the United Kingdom that a move towards a more managerial approach involving doctors has been marked by much stress as consultants have struggled with the duality involved in the role of consultant and clinical director. The need for a doctor to play the latter role is a matter of debate, but the need for all staff, professional and non-professional, to cope with their work being managed is a different and more universal requirement within modern health care. This is even more apparent in the community where the issue involves the novelty of working in a managed environment as well as the need to understand differently managed environments in order to work with staff within them. A case in point involves the increasing use of protocols to manage cross-boundary relations between agencies, and indeed between professions. Such devices have quite different implications in different settings, with highly bureaucratised structures seeing them as quite normal, and professional practitioners often seeing them as intrusive. Awareness of those differences would readily develop out of exposure to the wider array of organisational settings found in the community and should lead to greater sensitivity in protocol development.

ORGANISATIONAL TYPE

In community terms there are several issues which arise in relation to the type of agency involved whether statutory, voluntary, or private. This categorisation relates to issues of control, accountability, organisational and staff motivation and other features which are quite distinct in each kind of organisation. This is well illustrated in relationships between statutory and voluntary agencies where expectations of the latter often take little account of their part-time management, or the difficulties inherent in sustaining volunteer participation. Even between statutory agencies there are difficulties. In community care the processes of representative local government are often slow in order to allow for political accountability to be seen operating and this can be irksome to health authorities and professionals who experience fewer such constraints. Important questions are raised for professionals intending to work with, or within, such organisations.

These are not static features. In recent years some of these distinctions have become blurred with more agencies operating nearer to the boundary between categories, certainly in relation to their funding, and in relation to the kind of work with which they might be involved. This has been very clearly the case with the move to introduce tendering for public sector work and the implications for their organisation and accountability when voluntary agencies get such contracts. It is also apparent in the development of public–private partnerships where the attitudes within the sectors and their expectations differ so widely, but have to be submerged if they are to secure mutually beneficial opportunities. These arguments are relevant in all sectors of health care but they are particularly so within the community-based sector.

CLIENTELE AND ACCESSIBILITY

A key feature of organisations established to provide public services, or private services related to health, is the need for patient accessibility if they are to perform effectively. This is one of the key arguments in favour of community-based organisations which are often seen as having greater sensitivity and accessibility to their clienteles though a community base of itself does not guarantee this. Within the community setting many other organisational factors contribute to accessibility. Scale matters both in terms of the geography and the psychology of access, but more particular matters of location, organisation and formal and informal rules of access must also be taken into account.

Those apart, the nature of the relationship between clients and their service organisations is important, and varied. Formal registration of patients with a particular doctor, or practice, gives a continuity to the relationship which creates its own dynamics. Mutual learning becomes relevant over time both for patients and staff, and much discussion about changes in community-based care relates to that issue. Quite different, and much more like hospitals, are other agencies where contact is episodic and may be very infrequent. This is reinforced in cases like hospitals, or social service departments, where access is indirect and by referral, or at least where that is the conventional access route. The problem of dealing with direct referrals through, for example, hospital accident and emergency departments, illustrates the difficulties such institutions can face when conventional referral routes are not observed. Evidence that some of this direct patient demand may result from them being encouraged by community-based practitioners to refer themselves despite the impact this can have on hospitals illustrates the importance of this area. The reverse is also true. Open access to general practice can produce a complicated case-mix creating pressures which require careful management if they are to be reconciled with best practice. Changes in the organisation and management of hospital care can greatly amplify this situation through discharges from hospital which are often unplanned as far as the community side is concerned but which make immediate demands for care, often of a more complex kind than was traditionally required.

Issues of access, and of course of subsequent treatment, can become greatly exaggerated in agencies where there is formal public accountability, for example, through elections. Local government staff in the United Kingdom are used to elected councillors pursuing individual cases with professionals often having to comply with political demands as a result. There are signs of similar features appearing within health care. This can be further reinforced where patient, or public, participation in the organisation and delivery of care is established or simply encouraged. This has long been a characteristic of private care, where the patient, or the insurer, is more powerful than in a public system, and where quite different responses to patients characterise the systems. It is increasingly becoming a feature of public care in the guise of consumerism, or of patients' rights, or in the more extreme cases of patient control of services. The advent of such discussion and development in health care echoes earlier debates about housing and education where the implications of tenant and parent involvement are equally significant for professional and other staff work-ing in those areas (Boaden *et al.* 1982). Indeed, if such effects are not felt, there is a serious risk of participation being seen as merely symbolic with quite different, but equally serious, results. This consideration of client or public access and involvement with care provision links quite naturally with consideration of other non-agency ideas about community.

THE ANTHROPOLOGICAL VIEW

There are long-standing debates in fields other than medicine which are concerned with developing an awareness of, and an ability to work in and with, local communi-ties. In most of these cases, those involved do not have the ready inroad into the com-munity provided by well-established institutional health services which most local residents are used to using. Nor it should be said do they suffer the disadvantages which can arise from being an established service provider. Nevertheless they do have lessons to offer. This orientation to community reflects what Iliffe and Zwi refer to when they talk of the anthropological awareness involved in community-based med-ical education (1994). In some of the cases which will be reviewed later this approach is reflected in decisions to provide opportunities for students to be resident in local communities, sharing the experience of their lives with local residents and learning from that sharing. It echoes the more general assumptions which lay behind the development of the Settlement Movement in the late nineteenth century which pro-vided opportunities for the very elite university students of that time to gain a gener-alist exposure to the realities of life in communities which they would not otherwise experience. Such an approach may have considerable significance for the personal development of students, which was its original aim, while its professional relevance may be less direct but is no less important. It can also serve the purpose of develop-ing communication skills which are relevant in many communities in which profes-sionals will work but which are seriously conditioned when students arrive with their professional status and role already clearly defined.

This approach applies to a number of the curriculum schemes discussed later, and is much more evident in the developing world, or in more remote rural areas, where community-based experience is almost impossible without such residential opportunities. Even where such practical justifications are missing, there is an argument for resident experience which relates to the background of those usually recruited into medicine, but also to the wide differences of language and culture which occur in rural and urban communities. These features are just as relevant, often because they are less visible in the complex urban situations of developed countries. Such ideas about medical education echo the importation from the developing world of ideas about community development and how it could be facilitated in the United Kingdom and the United States in the 1960s and 1970s. These found their justification in the fact that professional community workers needed the skills necessary to work in and with communities to ameliorate and improve their circumstances and to alter the power imbalances which many communities experience in relation to professional institutions in developed countries. The relevance of such ideas in the health care context is somewhat ambiguous. On the one hand, medical services and some medical professionals were among those seen as problematic in many communities, while, on the other, many health care professionals would benefit from an awareness of those community development skills.

This is a radical conception of community-based education, however, especially in relation to medical education. There it is more common to see education delivered in quite varied settings but seldom with such radical agendas being involved. Much of the variety is simply a way of providing a vehicle for students to be attached to individual professionals practising different specialisms. The focus remains individual practice though some placements of this kind coincidentally give students an awareness of the wider agency setting or a professional's view of the community in which they are working.

SERVICE-BASED COMMUNITY EXPERIENCE

Health services

We discussed earlier the model of attachment to the individual general practitioner, or general practice, but there are a wide range of other medical agencies where attachment would provide useful broader experience and give another view of health care in the community. For example, it is common for GP trainees in the United Kingdom to spend some time with a community nurse and often to go out on home visits in the course of that attachment. The striking feature of that approach is the limitation of the experience, in terms of understanding the role of the community nurse, and the constraints and opportunities with which she works, and by comparison with the exposure to hospital clinical practice and to general practice involved in vocational training. If future models of care are to involve more collaboration across the professions, and especially if the doctor is to be the gatekeeper of access, or the manager of resource allocation to other community-based services, then it would seem that a wider early experience would be useful.

The same argument may be applied to a further range of organisations which might provide valuable educational settings. The increasing acceptance of alternative therapies, many beginning to enjoy wider popular acceptance, suggests one such set.

The array of lay-run, and locally managed voluntary agencies, dispensing health services in some form or other suggests another. The motivation for attachments and the potential learning involved in such placements would differ from conventional clinical experiences. Nevertheless both form an important part of the relevant wider community and students require extended and directed exposure to both if they are to understand properly their different roles, philosophies, constraints and activities.

Non-health services

A key point about the development of services within the community is that holistic ideas are encouraged, both in terms of treatment for individual patients and around wider issues related to the health of whole populations. As we saw earlier, these involve much wider relationships within medicine, or among health-related professions, than has traditionally been the case, but the argument for contact and shared experience during professional training extends well beyond such services. There is a wide range of other services offered within the community which are fundamental to people's economic and social well-being and which could be better integrated with health care (Boaden 1997). The most obvious case is social work where there is an overlap of professional interest and a recognition within the current system of the utility of such services and their ability to relieve the demands on health care. The list of relevant services can readily be extended to embrace counselling as a more formal skill, and some aspects of community psychiatric services might also fall in this non-medical category. Beyond this there are many sub-professional activities carried out by volunteers, or by paid staff within social service departments, all of which have direct relevance.

In all of these cases the same argument applies as did with earlier discussion. Full awareness of the agencies involved in such provision, and of the detailed work of their staff, will involve extended exposure to their work and experiential opportunities to work together in providing shared services. It is not enough to suggest that if they happen to be provided within the agency where training is located then they will be examined. It is a matter of securing access to them because they are relevant to a full understanding of the community and the services from which it might benefit.

This argument may be extended further to include a wide range of other organisations which are relevant. In formal institutional terms there are the housing and education services, whether in the form of the local authorities responsible for policy and wider provision, or in more local settings the housing associations providing social housing or individual locally managed schools. These are good examples of aspects of community life whose relevance for community health is widely understood and where learning opportunities could be mutually advantageous but where the institutional separation remains wide and frustrates development. There is an irony in the push for health education within health care where practitioners often struggle with educational processes and often lack the necessary skills while their teacher colleagues who have the relevant skills often treat health education as a marginal concern.

There are also the many voluntary groups and organisations which emerge in communities, resourced and organised in varied ways and providing key supports in relation to community health, whether for those who volunteer or for those they serve. Such organisations perform a range of key roles and the recent pressure on statutory services has tended to emphasise their role. This makes the relationship between such organisations more, rather than less, important and early training should address the significance of this aspect of community.

These varied aspects of organisations illustrate the range which is available in a typical community of reasonable scale and highlight the importance of seeking congruence between the setting chosen for community-based education and the aims and objectives being pursued. At its most simple this means that the established, conventional health care agencies are adequate to the task of producing doctors who will add an awareness of community-based medicine to their already adequate hospital-based capacities. At its most complex it means that the intending community-based practitioner may experience a wide range of organisational settings, and may extend their concept of the professional role to match the opportunities such a range provides. As we will see later, these different aims require different experiences within the varied settings and those experiences need to be timed and tailored to suit the stage of development reached by the trainee professional. This is readily illustrated by reference to some possible areas of professional work which extend beyond the traditional medical core.

Prevention, promotion and education

The significance of schools has been acknowledged in the last section, but education is much broader than that and many communities provide opportunities for their residents at all stages of life. Formal post-school education, both further and higher education, is one important and growing area but is often constrained in what it can offer by an increasingly vocational emphasis and by the economics of provision. These constraints may be less relevant in adult education where activity is often less formalised and established, but where costs are lower, opportunities often more widely available and where the less vocational aspects of community life may be engaged. This may form a fruitful area of partnership for health professionals concerned to develop health education and perhaps sensibly to avoid too close an association with established health care.

Similar arguments apply in relation to health prevention and promotion and are recognised among those active in such areas who have become almost another 'profession allied to medicine'. This creation of specialists may be a sign of established professions hiving off responsibilities in these areas, or in a more positive light it may be the key to developing the network of community relationships needed for this activity. Awareness of both those possibilities may be an important part of professional development and so needs to be engaged early in the community-based educational experience if it is to be seen as having more relevance in the professional career. Trainee professionals need to become aware, not that this is something they do not need to do, but that the community dynamics which surround advice sought, and taken, about health are important and they should learn how to tap into the established networks when the need arises. They need also to be aware of the social contexts in which behaviour patterns develop and the community constraints on behaviour rather than canvassing better individual behaviour against the grain of such community pressures.

ADVOCACY AND POLITICS

Less conventional than those established activities is the area of advocacy in relation to health and health care, and engagement with the political processes which affect both of them. These are not new areas but their range may well be extended as community-based health care develops in the future. There is already a highly developed politics associated with health in two areas. One is the representation of professional interests to government, and others, in relation to health care. This is an area where the profession has had much success, but where the politics have become more difficult and the competencies expected of the professional players have changed. The other area is in the field of public health where the specialist doctors do not treat patients and have relatively limited dealings with many of the direct providers of health care. Their key role lies in changing public behaviour, and in changing institutional behaviour in ways largely consistent with the prevention of ill health. They build on an established tradition from the nineteenth century in doing such work, but the focus of their influence demands high skills and understanding in relation to policy-making and decision-making and in the processes of institutional activity.

At one level the future for community-based care could lie in developing an enhanced capacity for relating to those public health professionals and responding to their demands for the evidence from which their influence might stem. Alternatively it might lie in the development of greater direct capacity among community-based practitioners to take on such roles themselves. In the United Kingdom the current ideas are for the development of collective action within primary care to shape health care delivery for large populations. Such activity will depend on skills which are not part of the current curriculum and which would benefit greatly from exposure to many organisational settings, but more particularly to varied people within such organisations. The dynamics of decision within organisations, and the timing of the decision process, are key elements in understanding what is decided, but also in having any potential influence over what is decided. This goes well beyond the personal call made on behalf of a single patient, and may in fact not be consistent with maintaining that approach to individual care. Change of policy may be a better goal than successful pursuit of a few individual cases, although that requires difficult decisions to be taken.

THE EVALUATIVE DISCIPLINES

Some of these 'new' tasks depend, as we saw in the last chapter, on the development of competence in relation to a range of new subjects which were characterised as evaluative disciplines. In some measure they depend on being introduced into the formal curriculum and will be taught alongside the established subjects in traditional ways. In addition, however, some of them do lend themselves to experiential reinforcement of learning, and to very abstract classroom teaching being leavened by real experience of such disciplines in use. The significance of some disciplines only becomes apparent when their purposes are clarified in this way.

Community settings are important to such opportunities and they will often be found outside traditional medical placements, or, if they are in health agencies, it may not be professional medical staff who are involved. Much decision-making in organisations is now made by specialist departments with finance and formal planning looming large in areas where in medical settings they might not traditionally have done so. More important in the context of disciplinary studies is the relevance to these specialist departments of disciplines such as economics and statistics, to say nothing of the management science which underpins basic organisational decisions in increasing numbers of cases. These are the settings where professional students might benefit from early exposure to other professions and semi-professions, and where there may also be some mutual benefit to be obtained from interaction.

In short, choosing the setting for learning is not simple nor are the many opportunities available easily exploited. As we shall see in later sections, sensitive use of the learning opportunities in the community will be a crucial factor in any development of community-based care which is to move beyond the current narrow professional focus.

6

Learning methods

Very broadly, methods used for learning in the community fall into two categories. The first covers all those techniques and methods suitable for classroom-based activity and include the lecture, small group work and case discussions. These can range from the didactic transmission of facts in a formal setting to highly interactive small group sessions or self-study using open learning materials or computer-managed learning resources. The second encompasses those whose principal purpose is to use experience as the basis for learning and includes clinical activities and those based on fieldwork within the broader community. Some methods used for learning in the community are not very different to those that may be used in the hospital setting, although the overall range of methods used is wider and the educational climate tends to reflect a closer teacher–learner relationship. In many instances methods used in the community could be used with effect in the setting of the hospital.

That this is not the case is a reflection of five factors. First, the organisation of teaching in the community is flatter and significantly less hierarchical than that of traditional hospital practice. Richard Horton writing in *The Lancet* about undergraduate medical education observes that 'Doctors are brought up to accept – if not always to respect – a hierarchical teaching environment: lecturers from academic faculty standing before packed rooms of drowsy students, or a senior physician imparting a distillation from a career's experience' (Horton 1998). In the teaching hospital setting organisation and tradition have conspired to distance the medical teacher from the medical student. Second, the personal style of many clinical teachers in the community encourages the development of a teacher–student relationship that reinforces an adult relationship between teacher and student. One consequence of this is that the relationship is generally closer and one-to-one meetings more frequent than is the case with ward-based teaching. This relationship fosters a learning climate that encourages discussion and exploration of issues that may sometimes be sensitive or related to personal attitudes and is rated very highly by students as one of the key features of their general practice attachments in conventional courses. Role modelling plays a very influential part in shaping attitudes to career choice, methods of study and towards fellow professionals (Haas & Shaffir 1982). However, there are dangers within such close relationships not least of which is the threat to the role-modelling element of clinical learning that the singularity of attachment to a limited number of community clinical teachers brings. Third, there is the influence of models of teaching used in vocational training for general practice that have been drawn very largely from adult education experience and that emphasise the importance of individual students concerns and expectations in the educational process. Fourth, lack of educational preparation for teaching in hospital implies that clinical teachers in that setting are likely to be unaware of the range of alternative methods that may be used for teaching. As a consequence, such teachers make use of a limited range of teaching skills. Finally, as we saw in the preceding chapter, the community offers a considerably wider breadth of settings for learning than the hospital, within many of which there are opportunities for addressing not just the bio-medical aspects of the syllabus but also psychological and social issues. This increases the likelihood of certain methods being used more often in this setting than in the relatively confined and structured hospital setting.

LEARNER-CENTRED METHODS

We indicated in Chapter 2 that there is a powerful trend in medical education towards actively involving students in the planning and implementing of their own learning. Such 'learner-centred' approaches are not new to other branches of health care education and examples may be found in, for example, occupational therapy education.

Neither are these approaches to education confined to the community setting with, for example, extensive use being made of the principles in postgraduate training for hospital practice in the United Kingdom (Parsell 1997). The decision to adopt learner-centred methods appears to reflect more the characteristics of the teacher rather than those of the learning context. Walklin (1990) defines such learning as those 'situations in which learners are expected, within reasonable limits, to take responsibility for identifying and agreeing objectives, planning and implementing their own learning activities and appraising outcomes with a tutor'. Courses based on such an approach encourage student activity and involvement by participation rather than solely didactic transmission of knowledge from teacher to student. Negotiated curricula and learning contracts are typical expressions of this approach to learning in higher and adult education and have been applied in community teaching with success in a variety of locations. Control of learning is shared between teacher and student with negotiation about which aims and objectives take priority, how content should be determined and chosen, and a preference for project-based and independent learning methods making wider use of resources being characteristic. Methods of recording learning include logbooks, portfolios and presentations of posters, reports and demonstrations, video and audiotape and oral discussions. The central learning activities in a community-based application of this approach focus on learning based on flexible experience in, and with, the community. Classroom-based learning still plays an important part and makes use of lectures, seminars, workshops and small group work. The emphasis in these activities is often on sharing information, explaining relationships, briefing and reflecting on learning activities, and broadening the participants' views through discussion, questions and debate. While outcomes are specified, they tend to emphasise application and use of knowledge over its acquisition using student behaviour as the principal assessment measure. Students are encouraged to think widely and reflect on their experiences and use them as the principal source of learning objectives and are treated as individuals with particular learning styles, preferences and priorities. Teachers using this approach to their teaching require a broad range of skills and play a number of roles – in stark contrast to the limited role of teachers in the traditional, teacher-centred, approach of conventional medical education. These skills and roles include establishing student learning needs and prior strengths and achievements, organising and resourcing learning activities, facilitating and enabling an appropriate learning climate, assessing achievement and providing feedback to the students about progress, evaluating learning sessions, effectiveness of the teacher and managing relationships and links with colleagues. There is also a need for involvement in planning, monitoring and controlling resources and playing a part in staff development.

In a recent example, Lennox and Pedersen from Leicester (1998) report a community-based multi-agency course organised for students in their fifth semester. The course was planned and implemented using learner-centred and problem-based principles and involved students in years 1 and 2 in the planning stage. A proposed structure for the course was drawn up by course planners and presented to student and staff committees and students in the tutorial group of one of the authors. The students chose preferred learning methods, prioritised sites to visit, commented constructively on the timetabling and evaluation arrangements, rejected the proposed group assessment scheme based on a case management plan and substituted their own ideas for individual plans on condition that they received help in their construction. Students worked in groups of three or four and interviewed patients, and the agencies involved in their care. Group members controlled group progress although experienced tutors were available for facilitation. Students used a workbook and a resource pack and each group generated unique sets of experiences. Assessment involved marking the case assignment in association with an external referee. Just under a third of the class received a grade of 'excellent' for their work. Student feedback about the course was very positive about all aspects and negative comments mainly reflected time constraints in the course.

Students themselves have expectations of their own for learning. Given a variable but not less than usually two-year period of socialisation into medical training before starting clinical work, it is not surprising that medical students should have narrowly focused ideas about the educational gains associated with an attachment to a general practice or community site. In a study by Stanley and Al-Shehri (1992) students in the fourth year of a conventional undergraduate course in the United Kingdom, identified their own learning objectives for a two-week attachment to local general practitioners. On average the students identified seven personal objectives. The accumulated class objectives were classified by content analysis into six themes. These included objectives focusing on the practice population and its health problems (e.g. epidemiology of common problems, social and background factors in illness); the role of the GP (e.g. difference between hospital and community practice, home visiting); the work of general practice (e.g. preventive care or immunisation); the management of general practice (e.g. the structure/organisation and finance of practice); general practice as a career (e.g. rules and regulations for training) and general learning objectives (e.g. consolidating existing knowledge and skills in other areas such as paediatrics, and seeing patients alone). The most frequently identified objectives related to understanding more about roles in community and primary care including relationships and team-working. Other commonly identified objectives included practising the skills of ear, eye and pelvic examination, improving communication and problem-analysis skills and learning more about prescribing and writing prescriptions.

Encouraging students to play a greater role in directing their own learning through their involvement in curriculum design or in the identification of learning objectives is an important step in helping them to learn the skills necessary for independent learning in their future clinical practice. Caution must be exercised, however, in determining the extent and timing of such involvement for two reasons. First, students must be able to regard such activities as meaningful, and second, students need sufficient experience and understanding to make the exercise professionally sensible within courses that are often of short duration.

PROBLEM-BASED LEARNING

One teaching method that has received considerable attention over recent years and that uses student-identified learning objectives as the driving force behind student motivation is problem-based learning (PBL). Problem-based learning and community-based learning are two closely linked concepts – so much so that some observers have considered it impossible to have one without the other. However, they are distinct and separate approaches to education in health care and it is worth exploring something of their individuality and the reasons for their proximity here.

Problem-based learning is a small group teaching strategy introduced by Howard Barrows and others to the teaching of medical students at McMaster medical school in Canada in the 1960s. Barrows developed the approach after concerns about student failure to transfer theoretical knowledge acquired in traditional lecture-based courses to the practical settings of the clinic and the ward (Barrows and Tamblyn 1980). Barrows was concerned about the importance of context in learning and of the need for students to learn to solve problems through analysing the issues and nature of information they required to progress. Considerable work on the nature of expert compared to novice thinking has been generated by his original ideas, and this has lead to new understanding about how clinical reasoning takes place and about the importance, not of inductive systematic reasoning as in the traditionally taught clinical systems history, but in the need to acquire and practise increasing numbers of 'scripts' concerning and describing ways of managing complex medical problems (Norman and Schmidt 1992).

In the original approach to problem-based learning students work on a clinical case presented on paper (although other media are now often used in addition). They work in sequence through possible responses to each step or stage in the presentation of the clinical case, and construct and justify questions to ask to seek out information that may help clarify the problem. As the case unfolds students make use of existing knowledge to progress but increasingly find they need to know more (or that their existing knowledge or understanding is inadequate). These learning needs or issues are listed on a blackboard and accumulate until the end of the session. The group discusses and prioritises these issues and agrees a group strategy for finding out about them in the interval (usually a few days) before the next session. This group 'learning contract' then forms the basis of the first part of the next session when each student reports back about what he or she has discovered through their period of independent learning. Through discussion guided by the tutor, students can compare what they know with their peers, and integrate their new understanding into their memory. They acquire and practise verbal argument skills and learn and make extensive use of many sources of information, including the Internet. They come to value the nature of information, its transience in a changing scientific world, and the importance of evaluating the evidence for, or against, an argument.

While the early forms of PBL were structured tutorials with the tutor playing an important guiding role, other variations have developed. Notably, in Europe at the medical school in Maastricht in the Netherlands, an approach that gives the students a considerably more prominent role in the overall process has emerged since the 1970s and is becoming more common throughout Europe, the United Kingdom and in Australia and the Far East. By following 'seven steps' (Box 6.1), students under the unobtrusive eye of the tutor work through the clinical case guided by a chairperson from their own group. Brainstorming plays a major role in developing ideas, engaging prior knowledge and in encouraging broad thinking around the problem. Characteristically, the problems unfold either during the tutorial session or over the course of a module – often following a real life case through a realistic course of disease.

PROFESSIONAL EDUCATION

A number of commentators (Eraut 1994; Taylor 1997) draw distinctions between education within the higher education sector and preparation for professional

---

Box 6.1 *The steps involved in problem-based learning*

- Clarify terms
- Analyse the problem by brainstorming
- Propose hypotheses or possible solutions
- Identify learning issues
- Carry out independent learning
- Report back and discuss newly acquired information in group
- Evaluate group and individual performance

practice in university settings. Such 'professional education' differs from higher education in a variety of characteristic, and for the teacher, quite fundamental ways. First, professional education especially in health care, exists in a state of dynamic tension with professional bodies and the professions, with the main employer (the NHS in the United Kingdom), and with government. Second, the curriculum addresses primarily the knowledge, skills and attitudes required for professional practice and this learning takes place not just within the setting of the university, but also in the context of clinical practice in the community and in hospital and other institutions. In addition, students who are engaged in learning in health care are motivated by a broad sense of ultimate career.

As we have previously discussed in some detail, it is very clear there are two certainties about the clinical context in which health care students, including medical graduates, will practise. These both have profound effects on curriculum and on the choice of teaching and learning strategies, teaching methods and resources, and crucially, on the methods of assessment used to cement the various links in the educational chain into place. These certainties are, first, that the world of clinical practice is changing and, second, that practice in the health service will increasingly rely on partnerships and collaboration both in providing clinical care at the bedside and in the community and in planning and commissioning such care. We will examine further aspects of these issues in some detail in the later chapters on inter-professional learning and on inter-agency work.

TRADITIONAL TEACHING MODELS

It is clearly intolerable that . . . we should continue at huge expense to train all doctors to be nascent specialists, and then retrain about half of them to be community generalists, only to find a gross shortfall in their performance of elementary tasks.

(Tudor Hart 1985, p.67)

A great deal of traditional medical education emphasises the transmission of information from teacher to student and the learning of clinical skills and attitudes by observing role models and 'experts' at work. Evidence has accumulated to demonstrate that this approach often leads to a superficial form of learning in which rote learning and memorising become the major learning strategies employed by students. In addition, there are concerns about the patchy nature of clinical skills teaching and supervision for individual students (McManus *et al.* 1998). The result is poor retention of factual detail over time and difficulty transferring information learned in a theoretical context to clinical applications. Students complain of stress related to the assessment system associated with such a memory-dependent system and about lack of choice and involvement with teachers. The more educationally desirable deep approach to learning encourages a search for understanding. Active involvement in learning, encouraging students to experience a need to know, providing opportunities for interaction with each other and with teachers through discussion (for example, in small group or problem-based learning) and the provision of a well-organised knowledge base related to other parts of the course are important elements that encourage such a deep approach.

Clinical education is largely based on observation of senior students or junior doctors at work in hospital with input from specialists and consultants in group settings such as classroom teaching, ward rounds and bedside teaching. Much individual learning with patients takes place at the bedside through 'clerking' exercises in which a systematic clinical history is obtained and an extensive clinical examination is carried out. The results of these clerking processes are then reported to more experienced staff through presentation at ward rounds or more formal teaching sessions. One danger of this unstructured approach is that it is possible for some students to see a clinical examination technique demonstrated once, practise it themselves and only have it assessed in the formal setting of an examination. There is considerable variation in the range of clinical cases seen by students within the hospital setting depending very largely on the nature of the 'firm' to which they are attached. As health care provision becomes more and more specialised within the hospital, general medical and general surgical attachments become more rare as attachments to breast cancer surgeons, invasive cardiologists, gastroenterologists, neurologists and neurosurgeons become more common. The medical and surgical specialities that have so much in common with the prevalence of disease in the community (dermatology, or psychiatry, for example) or with those techniques so much used by generalists (such as otoscopy and ophthalmoscopy) are sometimes referred to as the 'minor' specialities and are allocated correspondingly less time in the curriculum.

It may be detrimental to shift the balance of clinical education too far from an even mix between the hospital bedside experience and that of the community. Enthusiasts of the community approach argue that medical education for the larger proportion of graduates is ultimately aimed at producing general practitioners, therefore most clinical education should take place largely in the community, but it is important to recognise that benefits do accrue from retaining ward-based teaching on the menu. It is helpful to view the range of experiences available to students as a continuum (see Figure 6.1) with the choice of teaching or learning method based on the educational gains associated with their use at a particular point in the curriculum.

Hospital-based learning provides opportunities to care for, examine and manage patients with serious illness and to work with highly skilled members of other health care professions. It also offers opportunities to experience and learn from the

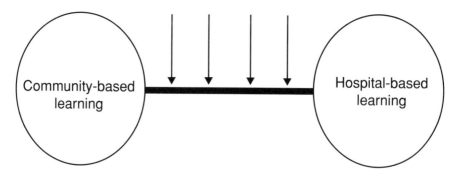

Figure 6.1 *The continuum of health care education*

atmosphere and climate of large clinical organisations by, for example, considering some of the managerial and administrative problems that such large organisations inevitably have and which impinge so heavily on health care provision. While traditional undergraduate education has very successfully made use of the clinical facilities of hospitals, little has been made of the opportunities for learning from and with members of the many teams operating within the setting, and even less has been made of the management opportunities. A report from the United States demonstrates this last point very well. Veloski and his colleagues (1996) in a recent study of medical student education in managed care settings, found that 16 per cent of medical schools required all students to have clerkship or other clinical exposure in a health maintenance organisation (HMO). The authors found that learning in these attachments very largely addressed clinical issues (often in the community or ambulatory setting) but did not address features unique to managed care such as cost containment or disease prevention. In fact, much of the learning that occurred was of the traditional clinical type and while it may have been assumed that other learning related to the setting of the clinical encounter, the HMO, was taking place, the authors argue that clearer objectives and more active management of learning is required to make effective use of the setting and the opportunities.

Inevitably, in a medical education system in which the production of young graduates capable of beginning a career as a pre-registration house officer (first-year intern) is the principal target, ward-based training is essential. This period of training has recently become the focus of intense academic and educational consideration in recognition of the need for this period to become more educationally meaningful to young doctors. Among suggestions for improvement in this year-long period are the greater use of educational mentors and learning contracts, better working and living conditions and a measure of competence at the end of the period. Greater clarity about the intended outcomes of the pre-registration year will help to more clearly define the educational aspect of this important period.

We have already discussed in Chapter 4 some of the aims and objectives of community-based education. These aims encompass a range of outcomes that include not only the understanding of the community as a social system in which people live and work but also as a location for learning to apply those clinical skills of history taking and clinical examination that are learned in hospital. In conventional undergraduate programmes such opportunities are rare, with attachments to general practice involving observation of the general practitioner and other health care workers at work. Over recent years there have been a series of successful experiments in teaching clinical skills in the community. Teaching in the community is receiving genuine support from general practitioners although issues such as time, financial reward and teacher training have still to be resolved (Gray and Fine 1997). Murray and colleagues (1995) identify six benefits of teaching basic clinical skills in the community. These are as follows:

- the wide range of common medical conditions and their accurate reflection of population morbidity;
- the opportunity to refine diagnostic skills by seeing large numbers of patients with undifferentiated problems;
- learning about chronic disease management;

- gaining an insight into the lives of patients thus understanding more of the inter-action between lifestyle and disease;
- close proximity to the uncertainty of medical practice;
- small teacher–learner ratios (typically 1:1 or 1:2) and prolonged contact hours with clinical teachers.

Teaching clinical skills to medical students has been the exclusive responsibility of hospital doctors for all of the twentieth century. Almost all of this teaching as we have seen, has been around the bedside of seriously ill patients in hospital although some teaching has been conducted in the out-patient department. The acquisition of his-tory taking and clinical examination skills has been a rather haphazard process of watching demonstrations, practising under widely varying levels of supervision and being examined formally in the 'Final' examinations. These examinations often con-sist of a 'long case' to test history taking, case presentation, clinical logic and exami-nation skills, and a series of shorter cases of typical lumps (hernias, tumours, etc.) enlarged organs (commonly the liver, spleen, or thyroid gland) in an attempt to provide some breadth. Candidates are only faced with similar situations in further, higher level, professional examinations, not in day-to-day professional practice, and especially not in clinical experience in the community.

The community element of many curricula has been increasing over the last ten years with especial emphasis on clinical skills teaching. Robinson and colleagues reported (1994) that half of all the academic departments of general practice in the United Kingdom were contributing to teaching basic clinical skills. To some extent this development has been a response to two factors. On the one hand, as we have seen in the introductory chapters, the hospital population is very different in recent years to that of the mid-part of the century. In particular in-patient stay times are much shorter and of those who remain in hospital, many are seriously ill or very frail. As a consequence, student clinical experience is dwindling (McManus et al. 1998) and alternative sites need to be found for teaching basic clinical skills. It is important to ensure that the skills taught at such sites are appropriate both to the site and to the part of the curriculum at which they occur. On the other hand, students have expressed dissatisfaction with traditional general practice attachments with one of the largest areas of discontent being the lack of practical skills teaching. Specifically, students have reported that their expectations of developing physical examination skills, taking cervical smears and giving injections are left largely unfulfilled by the end of general practice attachments (Lloyd and Rosenthal 1992). In the newer and more recently introduced teaching programmes, practice patients are used as teach-ing material with general practitioners as teachers. The organisation necessary to ensure a comprehensive mix of patients not withstanding the problems surrounding such problems of obtaining patients' consent, requires considerable amounts of time. One suggested option is the establishment of GP 'firms' whereby selected GPs pro-vide a similar form of clinical teaching to that provided on the hospital ward (Higgs and Jones 1995). This GP firm would replace a traditional attachment and would not only allow the opportunity to acquire and practise clinical skills in a range of com-munity settings, including the patient's home, but would also enhance the opportu-nity to observe continuity of care. As with the hospital firm, briefing and debriefing, feedback and assessment need to be incorporated to ensure the fulfilment of specific objectives. In addition, using a task-based framework, allocation of tasks during the placement could be used to link the experiences and skills gained to related topics in the wider curriculum. Greater use in teaching of GPs already attached to hospitals as clinical assistants has also been proposed bringing the potential for combined teaching with hospital colleagues (ibid.).

Another element of community learning consists of residential attachments of four or more weeks to a general practice surgery or health centre during the final year. The main goal of these attachments is to provide the student with an opportunity to experience everyday life in the community, in particular working alongside the GP and the primary care team, allowing for the practice of clinical skills in the community setting and the exposure to practice management skills. This relatively unusual type of attachment allows for students to be attached to remote practices and the opportunity to experience differing practice models.

Two recent papers from University College London describe the results and evaluation of an intensive clinical experience for medical students in general practitioners' surgeries. The papers are relatively unusual in that they describe both the evaluation of the project and the results of a randomised controlled trial of the effects of the attachments on student clinical performance. Such structured evidence comparing differing approaches to medical education is rare in the literature but essential to effective practice in education (Field and Kinmonth 1995).

After a four-week introductory course on clinical skills (history taking, basic physical examination techniques, communication skills and data interpretation) students in their first clinical year (the third year of a traditional medical course) were randomly divided into four groups. One of the groups spent five weeks in general practice and five weeks in hospital and changed over at the end of that period. The remaining three groups completed ten-week blocks in one of the traditional medicine, surgery, medical specialities and geriatrics and rheumatology junior rotations (Murray *et al.* 1997). The students' clinical skills were subsequently tested in structured clinical examinations at the middle and end of the attachments. The analysis focused on direct comparisons between the groups learning in general practice with those in hospital and on relative improvement over the second five-week arm of the study. Some 92 per cent of the class (208 students) took part in all measurements and no difference was found between students in either half of the rotations but those students who were taught in general practice improved slightly more than those taught in hospital. The authors concluded that 'students can learn clinical skills as well in general practice as in hospital' but recommended further work to clarify just which aspects of knowledge, skills and attitudes could be learned best in each site.

TYPES OF KNOWLEDGE

Methods of learning are inextricably bound up with the nature and context of what is to be learned. For professional education Eraut has identified and described three different forms of knowledge that underpin professional education. We have used this classification to cross-refer the discussion with examples of methods drawn from the literature in Table 6.1.

Table 6.1 *A classification of teaching methods in the community*

Type of knowledge		Site of learning		
		Classroom-based	**Clinically-based**	**Fieldwork-based**
Propositional	**Mode of use**			
	Replication *Application* *Interpretation* *Association*	lectures and other didactic input; self-assessment tests; CAL	observation of experts	attachments to community institutions and resources; collection of morbidity data; presentation of results of surveys
Personal		case discussion; ethics; role-play	role modelling inter-professional attachments	family placements; extended attachments to communities
Process				
	Acquiring information	case analysis; problem-solving exercises; study skills	observed or recorded consultations	data collection and analysis in the community
	Skilled behaviour	clinical skills centres	routine surgery sessions; observation; case analysis	
	Deliberative processes	small group problem-based sessions	shadowing senior and qualified colleagues	project work
	Giving information	communications skills courses	direct observation of consultations or recordings	presentation of reports; case studies; health promotion leaflets/posters; computer programmes
	Self-monitoring	small group work	reflection on practice	logbooks; audit projects; mentoring; learning contracts

The first category of knowledge, propositional knowledge, relates to the discipline-based concepts, generalisations, and principles that define practice and that can be applied in professional action. The second, personal knowledge relates to the interpretation of experience. In the health care professions where interpersonal relations are paramount to practice, personal knowledge has a direct bearing on practice.

Eraut divides the third element, process knowledge, into five types of process: acquiring information, skilled behaviour, deliberative processes, giving information, and controlling one's own behaviour.

Propositional knowledge

Propositional knowledge is the bedrock or 'core' content of a subject or discipline. It is the material used in the syllabus so often clearly set out in lists in course documents. For undergraduate medical education the propositional knowledge that is perhaps best known is that related to the basic sciences of anatomy, physiology and biochemistry, accompanied by elements of psychology and sociology in the early years. In later years the elements of pathology, microbiology, therapeutics and clinical differential diagnosis (commonly lists of signs and symptoms classified by disease) are included. A major problem with undergraduate teaching has been the almost inevitable manner in which students go about learning this 'core'. Because the method of delivery is usually a large class lecture and the method of examination is designed to test memory, often under extremes of pressure from volume of work, rote learning is the commonest mode of learning used with superficial recall as the result (Fransson 1977; Newble and Entwistle 1986). Eraut uses 'mode of use' as a way of sub-classifying propositional knowledge. These modes are replication, application, interpretation, and association. The replicative mode is the dominant form in higher education with students being presented with information that requires little or no reprocessing in their own minds before being used or tested. Application of knowledge involves making use of rules or procedures in novel settings or with new problems (as in problem-based learning), and interpretation involves an element of judgement based on choice and balance related to experience. Association involves the use of imagery or metaphors and is often intuitive, but can incorporate observation of others and subsequent integration of ideas or ways of doing into professional practice. Interpretation and application are major elements of professional practice and methods of teaching in postgraduate education, including for example random and problem-case analysis (Havelock *et al.* 1995). In this method doctors in training discuss in detail their management of a case with a more experienced supervisor.

What is the nature of the propositional knowledge associated with community-based education? We have seen from earlier chapters that the range of aims and objectives is broad but also that they differ significantly from the aims of clinical teaching in hospital. The 'evaluative' sciences of statistics, epidemiology, decision-analysis, health economics, ethics, and computer science have been mentioned earlier as elements additional to the basic traditional core of the bio-medical sciences and vital to the effective practice of medicine in the wider community-oriented health service. Later in this section we will use learning about management skills as an example of how some of these newer elements may be introduced into a curriculum.

Personal knowledge

Eraut's second category of professional knowledge is personal knowledge and the interpretation of evidence. He refers here to that knowledge acquired passively from experiences that are not overtly related to learning, especially those situations where 'trying to get things done' is the focus. Much of this knowledge is unprocessed and remains at what he calls the level of impression. This could include, for example, the student's passive understanding of the culture or atmosphere of a practice or clinic gained from watching and listening and taking part in day-to-day activities within a centre but not formally taught or discussed as a learning issue. Importantly, personal knowledge that is usually pre-propositional contributes significantly to the assumptions that people hold about their work and professional practice. It is one of the challenges for professional education to bring these assumptions into the open and to use them to explore the meaning of practice to the students and the context in which it takes place. Eraut writes:

> There are many experiences from which people learn without there being any intended educational purpose and without any codified, propositional knowledge being drawn to their attention. People naturally develop some constructs, perspectives and frames of reference which are essentially personal.

This knowledge then impinges on an individual student's view of practice, community and patients in the form of assumptions that are taken for granted and that are not either under critical control or processed and organised. This learning passively from experience also continues into professional practice, and students once they are aware of the importance of such experiences may learn how to deliberately make use of the learning potential involved. Personal knowledge is also gained through reflecting on the feelings that arise during learning experiences. Some methods of teaching, particularly role-play and the use of simulated patients, can give rise to strong feelings within students. Other sources of such emotions can include situations in which the students may develop strong feelings of attachment to patients. For example, intense feelings were aroused in a group of students whilst working with children who had been abused or neglected. The students developed apprehension about terminating their relationships with the children at the end of the project but with the help and support of the programme organisers were able to leave without feeling they were subjecting the children to another rejection (Schreier and Danilewitz 1989). This example highlights both the need for adequate briefing and debriefing of learning activities during which attitudes are challenged, and the central role that the tutor may play in supporting the student-learner.

The benefits claimed for extensive one-to-one teaching in the community include the early identification and solving of problems, encouragement of self-criticism and self-assessment, and encouragement of the student to 'take more responsibility for learning and feeding back their needs'. The sustained relationships between teacher and student in one-to-one teaching can play a crucial role in building the climate and opportunities for this kind of result.

Process knowledge

The third type of knowledge in the model is process knowledge. Process knowledge is at the heart of professional practice and makes great use of propositional (or 'content') knowledge. Process knowledge is 'knowing how' while propositional knowledge may be seen as 'knowing that': it is 'knowing how to conduct the various processes that contribute to professional action. This includes knowing how to access and make good use of propositional knowledge' (Eraut 1994, p.107). Five inter-dependent types of process are described, each of which has particular relevance to community-based education and are explored in detail below.

ACQUIRING INFORMATION

> The first object of any act of learning, over and beyond the pleasure it may give, is that it should serve us in the future. Learning should not only take us somewhere; it should allow us later to go further more easily.
>
> (Bruner 1960)

The search for and ordering of information are of course central to the role of the clinician. Learning how to take a history at the bedside, in the out-patient department and how to conduct a consultation in the surgery or clinic are cardinal aspects of medical teaching. The teaching of consultation skills has risen to prominence within vocational training for general practice both in the United Kingdom and the United States and features almost exclusively on the agendas of general practice trainers and course organisers in some parts of the United Kingdom. Models of the consultation vary but all rely on mastery of basic communication skills and differ from hospital-based history taking in their intention to reach a working hypothesis rather than conduct a broad-ranging enquiry. The effective acquisition of information relies on appropriate use of propositional knowledge and the selection of a suitable enquiry strategy. This means that students require a base of knowledge from which to start, at least an outline framework on which to shape the enquiry or questioning, and basic skills in collecting information. Interpretation of the information required relies on the building up of further propositional knowledge and sorting or filtering unimportant from important information. As experience builds up and the number of cases handled increases, students acquire 'scripts' for dealing with frequently occurring or serious conditions and these are integrated into propositional knowledge.

In considering the skills required for learning Eraut uses the classification described by Parker and Rubin (1966) to identify three processes necessary for academic study. These are:

- those that enable students to collect evidence, generate questions, observe, read and listen;
- those that allow the student to analyse, experiment, reorganise, integrate and consolidate information in order to make sense of it; and
- those that help the student to generalise and relate new knowledge to other situations.

In considering learning methods it is reasonable to go beyond those relating solely to learning about matters relating to content and clinical practice. Considering how students learn and how best to tailor teaching and learning methods to match the variation in learning styles and preferences is an important task for teachers. Ensuring that students acquire appropriate study skills and habits is another area where more work is required before we can be assured that students are making best use of all the opportunities available to them. Making greater use of learning methods that address each of the three general processes described above is one way of addressing this issue.

SKILLED BEHAVIOUR

In this context skilled behaviour means 'a complex sequence of actions which has become so routinised through practice and experience that it is performed almost automatically'. In addition to the performance of these daily professional tasks an element of rapid decision-making is also involved and these decisions are made generally at a sub-conscious or intuitive level in an interactive fashion with stimuli from the daily happenings of clinical work. It is clearly an advanced state that depends on the development of routines and is very difficult to break down into component elements and to change.

DELIBERATIVE PROCESSES

These are the processes that require combinations of propositional and contextually embedded knowledge as well as professional judgement such as those involved in planning, evaluating, analysing, and decision-making. Eraut proposes that certain conditions will characterise the situation in which these processes are invoked. These include conditions that are typical of encounters in the community and include: uncertain outcomes, underlying theory that is only partially helpful, inadequate knowledge about the context of the problem, pressure of time, a tendency to follow previous patterns of thinking and opportunities to consult with or refer to other people. In order to be effective, knowledge of the context and knowledge of practical courses of action and options are essential. This is the area in which adequate propositional knowledge in the fields of the evaluative sciences will be particularly effective in building up day-to-day skills in managing community-related issues such as the ability to handle health care information, manage resources, work as part of a team and integrate guidelines and protocols into regular practice.

GIVING INFORMATION

This refers to the ability to communicate with people at a level at which they understand and requires listening skills and the ability to use a commonly accessible form of language. Eraut draws attention to the 'teaching role' that this type of activity entails for the professional in the translation of propositional knowledge urbane to a profession into everyday information that can be understood and communicated to patients. For example, in the 'in-tray' exercise students work in pairs or trios to explain to each other in everyday language, the significance and routine management of common medical conditions. Students are encouraged to act as if they are speaking to a patient and, when using trios, the third student acts as observer providing feedback on the 'consultation'. There are many conditions that may be used and some commonly used ones include shingles, thrush, hypertension, scabies, boils, diabetes, asthma, obesity, smoking cessation, and the common cold.

DIRECTING ONE'S OWN BEHAVIOUR

Essentially this refers to the ability to be aware of what one is doing and why it is done in this way. In using the Argyris and Schön model of espoused theory to demonstrate the gap between what professionals do and what they think they are doing Eraut draws attention to the need for feedback (audit) on activities in practice.

DEVELOPMENT OF CLINICAL LEARNING

In describing the types of knowledge involved in professional learning we are considering one major element of the learning process and addressing the content of learning programmes. Such content is not acquired at once or simply, and there are chronological and programmatic influences both on how it is learned and on how it is used. Students may be seen to pass through a number of different stages as they learn in the clinical setting of the community and each stage has characteristic features that have implications for the type of teaching style adopted by the clinical supervisor and the nature of the learning experienced by the student.

Figure 6.2 shows in schematic form a model of educational stages involved in learning clinical skills in the community. While propositional knowledge is acquired variably throughout the course of community experience, this is most likely to be delivered in a classroom setting, for example, through concomitant problem-based learning activities. Usherwood *et al.* at the University of Sheffield describe an undergraduate course in which students spend six weeks on a general practice and public health module in their final year. The course is organised around two three-week attachments to local general practices and a weekly session of problem-based group work at the university (Usherwood *et al.* 1991). The group work is initially stimulated by a series of paper-based scenarios but students are encouraged to 'regard the experiences of their practice attachments as providing legitimate problems for discussion upon which to base their learning contracts and subsequent presentations back to the group' (ibid., p.428). Learning resources include literature and other library facilities, a patient interviewing course including video recordings with patients from their practices, a visit to a local hospice for the dying, local teachers and practice staff and their GP teachers. Assessment methods include criterion-referenced profiles, a computer-simulated surgery and a video recording of a consultation.

Process and personal knowledge are addressed and consolidated through learning from the experiences provided in the community and it is one of the prime responsibilities of the teacher to ensure that this is adequately incorporated into the practice and behaviour of the student. Each stage of the model has discrete elements of its own but there is scope for considerable overlap in some of the areas described depending on clinical and educational circumstances (Deutsch 1997).

Stage I Exploration

In this first phase, students are at the beginning of their experience of the community as a setting for clinical work. Generally as we have seen, they arrive from a profession-

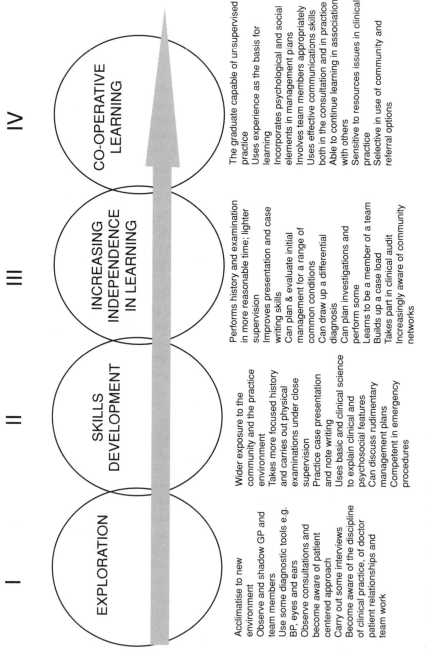

Figure 6.2 *Phases of learning in the community*

specific background often in the first or second year of their undergraduate experience. Typically in this early community experience, they will observe the work of the general practitioner and other members of the primary care team, in particular the nurse and practice staff. The time spent on attachments such as these is often limited (for example, a day a week in the second semester) and is a small part of a general educational climate that concentrates on basic science teaching in the academic setting of the medical school. Student expectations in these circumstances relate to exploring the role of the GP and the practice, seeing the range of clinical material that passes through a surgery and talking to patients about their illness experiences (for example, the objectives identified by students in Stanley and Al-Shehri 1992). There are chances to practise some basic clinical skills (often for the first time), for example, taking blood pressure, listening to the chest or examining the ears. Opportunities to interview selected patients, sit in the waiting room, work with reception office staff and travelling with the clinician supervisor on home visits and other activities are common. The close contact on a regular basis with their supervisor and the practice environment provides opportunities to think about and discuss the nature of medical practice in the community, the patient-centred approach to the consultation and the varying levels of uncertainty that surround clinical decision-making. The roles and responsibilities of the other members of the health care team become apparent for the first time and the range and diversity of patient demand can be explored and analysed against the background of the students' own experiences and initial grounding in the principles of epidemiology. The clinical and social issues presented by patients also raise moral and ethical issues and these bring a broader dimension to the experience. These early experiences in the community can also involve attachments to families for more intensive study, for example, students may be attached to families with a new or soon expected baby (Pill and Tapper Jones 1993).

Stage II Skills Development

The next stage in the developmental process marks the beginning of the process through which the student takes increasing responsibility for his or her own clinical actions. At this early stage the student is entirely dependent on the clinical teacher and the degree of clinical supervision is very high. During this phase students gain wider exposure to the practice and its setting in the community. In the example from Lennox and Pederson (1998) students interviewed agencies involved in the care of selected patients to gain a deeper insight into the relationships and roles played by each in the care of chronic conditions. In the practice, clinical learning continues with students taking more focused histories and carrying out appropriate physical examinations, applying under close supervision clinical skills learned initially in the setting of a clinical skills resource centre or at the bedside in hospital. There are opportunities to learn and practise the important skills of clinical record keeping and of case presentation and of discussing options for patient management, especially for the more common conditions. At this point in the curriculum, students are largely unaware of the details of pathology that may explain the problems presented to them. This offers excellent opportunities for the application of the underlying principles of the natural sciences of anatomy, physiology, biochemistry and those of psychology and sociology, to analysing the clinical problem. These problems may subsequently be used as the basis for further small group learning. Because students are intimately involved in the work of the practice at least for part of the working day, they may be exposed to a range of clinical circumstances including potentially life-threatening ones and a number of medical schools are ensuring that students are competent in the elements of basic life-support before they take part in clinical practice.

Stage III Increasing independence

At a later stage in the curriculum, typically years 4 and 5, students can move on to perform history and physical examinations in more reasonable times. They begin to build up a 'case load' of patients or families whom they see regularly – an important step in learning about the value of continuity and long-term care that are central tenets of community practice. Presentation and case writing skills are enhanced, and students can play a significant part in drawing up a differential diagnosis and management plan for the common range of community morbidity. Playing a role in the management of patients naturally raises opportunities for consideration of team-working issues such as the roles and responsibilities of team members, communication skills within a team and the organisational and administrative issues involved in the diffuse setting of a practice. Once a reasonable number of clinical cases have been seen by the students it will be possible to collate details and plan audit projects based on morbidity recording and clinical management principles. This leads on to consideration of the importance of clinical protocols and the use of evidence-based sources and information technology in the support of clinical decision-making. The student by now has begun to study pathology and the other clinical science disciplines including microbiology, chemical pathology, medicine, surgery, paediatrics, obstetrics and psychiatry. The community experience provides opportunities to integrate learning in these areas into consideration of the problems presented in clinical practice. The role of the clinical supervisor in this phase has three elements: first, to provide adequate exposure to clinical conditions in the community and to provide observation and feedback of the use of history and physical examination skills; second, to ensure the student has opportunities to integrate learning in the community with other aspects of the curriculum, including hospital- and classroom-based learning activities; and third, to act as personal mentor and guide to the young clinician during what is a long period of sustained contact.

Cooperative learning

A fourth stage of cooperative learning is reached when experience is the main basis for learning typically in the pre-registration and vocational training periods. We will return to this stage later in the book.

The model describes the nature of the relationship between teacher and learner moving from one of dependence in the early undergraduate years through a stage of increasing independence during late clerkship and early post-qualification experience to one of cooperative learning in which both teacher and learner share responsibility for the learning process (including assessment) and evaluation of its effectiveness. The learning contract is a useful vehicle for recording and monitoring learning at this stage and has been used widely in vocational training for general practice and in hospital-based training in the postgraduate years (Parsell and Bligh 1998).

The model shown in Figure 6.2 suggests that the first three phases are separated from the fourth and in most courses this is the case. The organisation and delivery of undergraduate medical education are separate from the organisation and delivery of vocational training for general practice and almost completely unrelated to postgraduate preparation for hospital specialist careers. One approach to correcting this lack of curriculum continuity has been described at the University of Illinois. This programme for primary care not only addresses the need for a link between the various years of the undergraduate programme to provide a coherent learning experience but it also reflects the three elements of professional knowledge described in Eraut's model of professional development.

Case studies

The Longitudinal Primary Care (LPC) program for undergraduate students at the University of Illinois at Chicago's College of Medicine was introduced as an initial step in overall curriculum reform towards a community-based framework for a large (by US standards) annual intake of 180 students (Freeman *et al.* 1995). The LPC program is a three-year course that starts in first year. Students are attached to a preceptor clinician drawn from family medicine, general internal medicine or paediatrics and spend between half a day a month in year 1 and a half-day a week in year 3 with the teacher. Year 1 focuses on interviewing skills and students learn about the 'meaning of illness to the patient in the context of the patient's family, community, and culture', thus addressing both propositional and personal knowledge while providing a firm input to process knowledge through learning techniques of history taking. In year 2, students begin to develop a panel of patients and learn about the use of community resources and risk assessment. In year 3, continuity of care emphasising relationships over time and team-work in health care are the major learning issues in weekly half-day attachments. Syllabus content is based on the 20 most commonly occurring conditions in primary care in the United States. The program is voluntary but after some three years has developed from a starting group of 54 selected students to a busy 160 students and 140 preceptor sites.

A further step has been taken at Case Western Reserve University in Cleveland and Detroit in response to the Robert Wood Johnson Foundation's Generalist Physician Initiative (GPI). The GPI is a $32.7 million grant programme that challenges medical schools in the United States to collaborate with state governments, private health insurers, health maintenance organisations, hospitals and community health centres to increase the production of generalist physicians. Some 86 medical schools applied for support, 18 were selected to receive 18-month planning grants and in 1994, 14 six-year implementation grants were made to 16 schools to help them increase the number of graduates entering a generalist career. As an example of one of the initiatives, Case Western School of Medicine collaborated with the Henry Ford Health System to develop a seven-year combined medical school and residency curriculum for primary care. One of the main goals of this ambitious programme is to provide the skills and attitudes required for leading further change in the movement towards generalist physicians in the United States in the future. The primary care course extends from admission through to the residency programme for graduates. Only the early elements of the course have been designed so far but already it is possible to see the introduction of some elements of the evaluative sciences that will form the basis of the propositional knowledge of community practitioners in the future. In the first year these include managed care, health economics, advocacy, the value system of generalist practice and the organisation of health care. In the third year clinical learning is in integrated blocks that address four broad domains that reflect the way patients receive care rather than the more conventional curriculum organisation based on departments, and include health maintenance and disease prevention, primary and emergency care, tertiary care and rehabilitation. Each student has a clinical base in a community practice and attends regularly starting as observers but moving quickly on to taking responsibility for clinical history and physical examinations. A personal learning plan and a personal adviser/advocate system lie at the heart of the educational process and ensure the course is responsive to student needs and requirements.

These curriculum initiatives address the extension of undergraduate medical teaching into the community. Like the UK examples from Leicester and London they focus on providing appropriate settings for students to learn about clinical skills and to explore something of the atmosphere and culture of community clinical practice. However, they are all centred on an experience that is essentially medical/clinical in their focus. The teaching methods employed vary from those used in hospital in the attention paid to the student but the content is broadly similar. The community offers much more both in learning opportunities and in providing a context for future practice.

HEALTH SERVICE MANAGEMENT

For tomorrow's doctors to be competent in their professional lives in a culture that values accountability and flexibility they will require skills additional to those traditionally acquired in clinical courses. These skills will involve, at their core, the ability to work within a managed service and, for some, skills required for being involved in management itself. But it will be necessary not only to work within a managed system but also to be able to influence it and develop within it as a professional. The advocacy role played by clinicians on behalf of their patients also requires considerable understanding of the structure, organisation and the dynamics of the health management system. The active involvement of the public health element of the community clinician's work requires skills and understanding in areas such as data management, public relations, critical analysis, and written communication. Then there are the technical aspects of subjects well removed from the common core of bio-medical syllabuses, for example, health economics. While almost every practising clinician in both the United States and the United Kingdom will be aware of the terms opportunity cost, or cost-benefit analysis, just how secure are we when it comes to applying the principles behind the terms to everyday clinical practice? These areas of organisational structure, political science, and economics are neither taught nor learned in most undergraduate courses. But they are clearly important if not crucial, to the effective practise of population-based medicine. How should they be introduced into a curriculum and what methods might be used to address them?

Very few conventional undergraduate courses will offer curriculum time to the area of health service management (other than outline talks about the organisational map) often seeing it as largely irrelevant at the early stage of a student's career and preferring to postpone exposure, if any, to the postgraduate years (Foreman 1986; Petersdorf and Turner 1995). This approach essentially guarantees that students will not gain any experience of management, the largest and most important determinant of health service delivery. But say it was possible to introduce teaching about how the health service is organised and managed, how would it be possible to organise the curriculum so that the educational principles of relevance, meaning, active involvement, progressive learning and optional learning around supplementary material are all respected? One way of achieving this is not to invent new learning methods but to make best and imaginative use of the already tried and tested classroom, clinical and fieldwork methods we have already discussed.

Fairhurst et al. (1995) draw a comparison between clinical generalist skills of information gathering, broad analysis of problems, and shared decision-making with those required in general management, especially when handling undifferentiated problems. They argue that medical students must learn to manage their own learning and in time, their own clinical practice, so it is most appropriate that they also learn the principles and skills required of management. They suggest that the propositional and process knowledge in this area will include an understanding of corporate governance, team building and leadership. Learning methods should build on existing skills (e.g. of time management or prioritisation) and stimulate motivation and self-study in the early stages. Later, through the use of task-based activities students can engage in academic and service-related issues by applying more sophisticated skills such as negotiation, presentation, delegation and task analysis in the management of more complex problems.

We saw earlier that understanding organisations was an important aspect of modern clinical practice. The need to work within a managed environment and the need to understand such environments was raised and the differing perceptions of manager and clinician to the use of protocols used to highlight the point that much stress can result from a mismatch of expectation and experience. We felt it was important to develop appropriate levels of awareness amongst health care professionals by, for example, exposure to a wider range of organisational settings. According to Cohen (1995) the educational implications that arise from working in highly managed clinical environments include learning to manage resources through the results of health service research, taking part in the development of clinical guidelines, understanding clinical epidemiology, using evidence to support decision-making, working as a team member and practising as a professional. As Veloski (1996) and his colleagues have shown, concerns that many US medical schools are not altering their teaching programmes to adapt to the needs of graduates who are likely to practise in HMOs are important. It is estimated that between 45 per cent and 60 per cent of the United States will be covered by some form of managed care programme in the next ten years (Meyer et al. 1997).

Meyer and his colleagues carried out a survey of all 125 medical schools in the

United States in 1995 to define a core curriculum appropriate to graduates working in a managed care service. They found that of the 91 schools responding, the majority claimed to have or to be planning relevant programmes, although much of the teaching reflected either existing material or was based largely in the classroom setting. Using focus groups of administrators and clinicians from a managed care background they identified and prioritised the skills and knowledge they felt should be included in study programmes and a clear consensus emerged around a common core of material.

We have used parts of this core curriculum to design a hypothetical curriculum for undergraduate medical students (Table 6.2) that draws on standard teaching and learning methods. This programme would fit well into a number of recently described courses, for example, the new curriculum at Case Western with its longitudinal commitment to the continuous curriculum, or our own problem-based undergraduate course in Liverpool. It is a way of introducing new and highly relevant material into a student-learning environment in a way that mirrors other subjects. It also integrates with other learning and stimulates the students to apply what they already know to examining how a system that is crucially important to their future professional lives works. The novel learning method, role-play of a health service management board, is based on similar methods used extensively in management training. Such games are highly motivating for participants, they challenge existing beliefs and require active participation and independent learning to complete. They

Table 6.2 *An outline of possible content and methods for an undergraduate curriculum in health service management*

	Method	Content
Year 1	Small group problem analysis of case study material, supported by didactic input, guided reading, case presentations and attachments to managers at local Health Authorities/HMOs	Biostatistics, decision analysis, economics, law, ethics, IT, communication skills, principles of management (e.g. time management)
Years 2 and 3	Role-play exercises simulating health authority management boards dealing with common problems, e.g. resource allocation decisions; continued attachments	Communication skills (e.g. negotiation), team-working, decision analysis, clinical epidemiology, IT
Year 4	More complex/in-depth case studies supported by practical project work, e.g. setting up a community screening clinic, dealing with complaints or handling an epidemic; longer elective attachments	Ethics, law, communication skills (e.g. delegation), team-working, risk management, quality assurance, population issues, economics, task analysis, IT, project planning
Year 5	Shadowing service managers in e.g. budget setting or policy planning activities	Communication skills, politics, utilisation and risk management, managed care, team building, public relations, project management

lend themselves to small group work but require considerable preparation in the early stages especially in writing the case study materials. However, once this is done the role-play is free-standing, needing only occasional revision. It will be very difficult for many medical teachers to prepare such materials without close collaboration with health service managers and management consultants involved in training. This collaboration is not likely to be a bad thing as it brings a high degree of mutual understanding to all involved during the working together process. The remainder of the outline follows the traditional teaching pathway of the early introduction to the terminology and principles of the subject often, and conveniently, delivered in classroom settings of small group work and didactic input followed by increasing exposure to practical issues through role-play or projects and completed by assessment of learning using appropriate methods.

The learning methods are not new but the content and the setting are. This gives rise to concerns about a common problem in professional, and especially medical, education – the amount of influence exerted by existing teachers (or sometimes the educational climate) on the student when new ideas are introduced into a teaching programme. It is not appropriate to review here the arguments surrounding the 'hidden' curriculum that lies within any programme of teaching and learning, but it is appropriate to discuss the particular effect that often strongly held individual views about other health care professions (and managers may be counted amongst these for the purposes of this argument) may have on the students' perception of the importance of learning. It would not be overstating the case to say that there is a dynamic tension between clinicians and managers within the health service. This tension is not new but has gathered force in the last decade as changes to the organisation and funding of the health services both in the United States and the United Kingdom have given prominence to the role of general management in both countries.

CONCLUSION

In this section we have examined various methods for learning in the community in the light of recommendations for curriculum change, and changes to clinical practice consequent to demographic, scientific and political pressures. Different types of knowledge, propositional, personal and process, appropriate to professional education have been defined and examples given of how learning methods might be used to stimulate students to learn within these areas.

There is some debate over the nature and substance of the propositional knowledge that will form the 'core' of community-based education. There are attempts to reposition old material into more appropriate parts of the continuum of medical education by moving some elements into postgraduate training and discarding other less relevant or out-of-date ideas. New material is waiting to be introduced including those elements of the evaluative sciences discussed earlier. It is important, of course, not to move from the one extreme of a bio-medically overloaded curriculum to another that is packed tight with psycho-social material leaving the student with just as much work to do. It is, however, in the realms of personal and process knowledge that most progress will be made in addressing modern medical education to the needs of clinical practice in the early twenty-first century. This will be characterised by collaborative practice, team-working, a clinical focus on promoting health within individuals and in populations, and continuing emphasis on the effective and efficient management of resources. While some of the methods described above carry considerable potential for effective learning in these areas, they are currently solely focused on the acquisition of clinical attributes relevant to the conventional model of medical practice. We will see in Chapter 7 addressing inter-professional learning that problem-based small group work and shared clinical experience in caring for patients can be used with effect by students from a variety of health care backgrounds to learn about not just their own professional concerns but also about each other's roles and beliefs. But gaining insights into the work of other members of the health care team is unlikely to be sufficient preparation for a lifetime of practice in the wider and more complex community in which graduates of today's education system will practise. It will also be important to be aware of the political and organisational structures (and the dynamics of their relationships) that combine to make the modern health care system work, and to understand the huge range of services and providers of care in the community that fall within the non-statutory and voluntary sectors.

7

Inter-professional education

We have so far looked closely at some of the style and characteristics of medical education at undergraduate level. We have also considered broader aspects of education for the health care professions. These have included the use of a wider range of sites for learning and the incorporation into the curriculum of subject matter more relevant to practice in managed health care services. Doctors no longer practise alone or in isolation from their clinical colleagues. Modern health care is delivered by teams of professionals both in hospital and, especially, in the community. In this chapter we look at examples of how some health care professionals are being prepared for a clinical career that is increasingly team-based and consider some examples of innovative ideas for teaching. Some of the implications for education in the future, including team-based learning, will be raised. But first it is worth considering some of the contextual matters that influence the need for and the setting of inter-professional education.

We have suggested that there is a need for a closer relationship between educational developments in health care and policy intentions within the NHS. It is not just within the United Kingdom that there have been profound changes in the management and organisation of health care. Moves towards greater use of primary care as the leading edge of national health care delivery can be traced back for a considerable time. A major part of the World Health Organisation's thrust towards worldwide health reform during the late 1980s were demands for radical changes to the site and character of health care education. Concerns that existing curricula failed to address patients' needs, concentrated too much on hospital-based care and did little to favour team-work between health personnel were reflected in the Edinburgh Declaration issued by the World Federation for Medical Education in 1988. Among the twelve Principles set out in this Declaration, there was a clear call for educational activities stimulating and developing team-work among those who would work together in the health services, and especially those in primary health care (Box 7.1).

Box 7.1 *The Edinburgh Declaration 1988*

The Twelve Principles

1. Widening of educational settings.
2. Using national health priorities as the context for education.
3. Active learning throughout professional life with appropriate reforms to the assessment system.
4. Professional competence as the purpose for all learning.
5. Training the teachers as educators.
6. Health promotion and disease prevention to feature strongly.
7. Integration of science into clinical practice.
8. Selection of entrants for non-cognitive as well as cognitive abilities.
9. Coordination of education with health care delivery services.
10. Balanced production of doctors to meet national needs.
11. Increase the opportunity for joint learning, research and service with other health and health-related professions, as part of the training for team-work.
12. Recognising continuing professional development as the main sphere of medical education.

In the United Kingdom, the NHSME (National Health Service Management Executive) in its policy statement concerning nursing in primary care (1993) drew particular attention to the crucial part that team-working will play if health and social care in local communities were to be of the highest quality. Surprisingly, given the emphasis placed on such moves, the establishment of multiprofessional learning at undergraduate level has been subject to considerable difficulties despite there being a long history of such education at postgraduate and continuing education levels (Areskog 1988). While it is likely that organisational factors are prominent in causing some of the difficulties in implementation, the attitudes and skills of health care teachers and managers must also play a part. Engel refers to the '*political will* that will be necessary to provide the motivation, facilities and resources essential for genuine, sustained collaboration' (Engel 1994).

Integrated provision and shared professional care are likely to be among the main hallmarks of the future primary care. This dual set of changes puts enormous pressure on medical education to produce doctors capable of working effectively, and of continuing to learn, in this essentially novel, for them, environment. While for nurses, social workers, and health visitors, multiprofessional working environments are not new, medical training has striven to retain a fierce separation from the contamination of ideas such as team-work. Maintaining autonomy and the status quo of past working conditions may be seen as one of the outcomes of traditional medical education (Tope 1996). Health care professionals working in the primary care of the future will need to react to change and adapt to broader roles and relationships. The effectiveness of health care education in the future will be dependent on both the nature and the form of the education provided and the opportunities and constraints of the realities of practice. Interdisciplinary team-work is a complex and dynamic cluster of relationships that needs to embrace a very broad range of skills and attitudes.

SOME DEFINITIONS

Shared learning among the health care professions goes under a number of different names. These are often used interchangeably when describing the array of activities available to both undergraduates and postgraduates. It is helpful to standardise the terms used when describing educational activities at least so that the reader knows that like is being compared with like. In this book we use inter-professional learning to mean learning activities involving two different professional groups, for example, nurses and doctors or medical students. Multiprofessional learning means activities in which more than two groups learn together, for example, nurses, doctors and social workers. By interdisciplinary learning we mean learning activities that involve two branches of one profession, for example, midwives and health visitors, or junior hospital doctors and registrars in general practice. Multi-disciplinary learning therefore refers to learning activities involving three or more branches of one profession, for example, practice nurses, midwives and health visitors.

PURPOSES OF INTER-PROFESSIONAL LEARNING

There is little disagreement that a major rationale for inter-professional education relates to the need for professionals who work together to gain an understanding of each other's knowledge and skills. Knowing what others know and what they can do helps to shape and form attitudes and reduces prejudice. The ultimate prize for success in such educational activities is likely to be better patient care (Jones 1986). But not only is it important for members of health care teams to be aware of each other's professional strengths and weaknesses, it is also important that they can work as members of a team. So a second aim of inter-professional learning is the acquisition of effective team-working skills. The increased awareness gained through learning together should then help individual professionals to make best use of their colleagues, improve communication, assist in sharing of tasks, and lead to appropriate delegation, sharing of responsibility and the more effective use of leadership skills. Similarly, it is not unusual to find that inter-professional educational activities aim to help participants find shared values and develop new perceptions of each other's professional viewpoint (Jones 1986).

SETTING OF INTER-PROFESSIONAL LEARNING

Much contemporary teaching is undertaken in large group settings such as the lecture or large discussion group. Often these settings combine the economic benefits of size with the disadvantages of anonymity and homogeneity of identity. It is now clear from a number of sources that such large mixed classes are unproductive, often result in student groups ignoring one another and can lead to feelings of resentment that learning opportunities are being somehow diluted (Szasz 1969). Students prefer to work on problem-solving tasks in a cooperative atmosphere, for example in pairs, trios or small groups rather than in these larger settings (Areskog 1992; Szasz 1969; Carpenter 1995).

NEW APPROACHES TO THE UNDERGRADUATE MEDICAL CURRICULUM IN THE UNITED KINGDOM

To what extent does undergraduate medical education, especially in the UK, prepare medical students for this world of team-work? What opportunities are there for shared learning, and for working together with students from other health care professions during the undergraduate experience?

Tomorrow's doctors

Recent and continuing changes in medical education are having wide-ranging effects on the preparation of medical students for a career in the NHS. As we have seen in earlier chapters, these changes include a greater use of small, problem-based group work, and the earlier introduction of clinical skills teaching. They also aim to prepare doctors for a lifetime of continuing learning and professional development. The architects of this change have long recognised the need to release doctors from the shackles of their undergraduate education and to prepare them for a career in which knowledge is constantly changing and in which no single profession is paramount. While much of the change currently visible is related to improving the learning environment by, for example, reducing the factual overload so characteristic of traditional undergraduate medical programmes, there are also less obvious attempts to improve the process through which students learn. These include changes to the educational climate towards a student-centred learning environment where the vocational character of medical education is established at an early stage. Changes to the system of assessment to emphasise the importance of clinical and communication skills and the use of knowledge in problem-solving rather than the use of memory recall skills will also make significant impact on the ways in which students learn. Crucially, there is also recognition of the 'training' effect that years of traditional lecture-based teaching can have. The introduction of special study modules into the curriculum for all medical students provides an excellent opportunity for ensuring that the university experience for doctors of the future contains a broader element of 'education' that can release and stimulate individual interests and foster a depth of learning previously reserved for those undertaking intercalated degrees. The list below shows a selection of the four-week special study modules available to year one students at the medical school at the University of Liverpool.

- Genetic engineering and biotechnology
- Screening for cognitive impairment
- Complementary therapies
- Membrane biology – the internal environment
- Life cycle of a nerve cell
- Occupational therapy

- Caring for neurological disease
- Drugs for tropical disease
- Follow that pathologist!
- Heart failure in the elderly

It is notable that on the menu is a module on occupational therapy. In this module 12 students worked for four weeks alongside occupational therapists and their clients (Tyldesley and Green 1997).

As we saw in the last chapter, medical students are taught in a pattern of two years of introduction to the basic sciences of anatomy, biochemistry, and physiology and to the behavioural sciences of psychology and sociology. This 'preclinical' period is followed by three years of largely hospital-based clinical studies. Such courses tend to be based on lectures and practical classes in the early years followed by ward-based teaching of clinical history taking and examination supervised by hospital specialists. As with other health care professions, medical students are trained in a protected professional environment within the medical school, so that contact with students in related professional groups, nurses, physiotherapists, pharmacists or social workers, let alone students in the wider university setting, is kept to a minimum (Chastonay 1996). Ward-based teaching is a period of intense socialisation for many students that often comes as a surprise and a challenge after two years of conventional teaching in the narrow confines of the medical school (Haas and Shaffir 1982).

While there are emerging opportunities then for shared learning activities at undergraduate level, there are few examples of good practice in the literature. There are reports of shared teaching at postgraduate level and in a series of national surveys the Centre for Advancement of Inter-professional Education (Barr 1994; Barr and Waterton 1996) found that while many of these activities attracted a broad range of health professionals, they very rarely involved doctors. It is also clear that descriptions of courses are more common than evaluations of their effectiveness. The gathering and presentation of evidence are of increasing importance in a clinical world that looks towards evidence-based practice as the gold standard, and of considerable importance when considering the financial and human resource issues involved in introducing or extending multiprofessional learning. Without the evidence for its effectiveness these arguments are thin and difficult to defend. There is, however, some controversy about how best this evidence can be collected. On the one hand, some researchers argue that the nature of the educational aims in inter-professional learning is such that qualitative data collection and analysis methods are most appropriate. Such methodologies include interviews, focus groups, diary surveys, observational techniques and purposive sampling techniques. On the other hand, there is a rising call for evidence based on quantitative methods, and in particular the biomedical 'gold standard' the randomised controlled trial. In a recent paper, Zwarenstein and colleagues (Zwarenstein 1997) described their progress on a systematic review of evaluation of the effectiveness of inter-professional learning. After setting a minimum number of methodological requirements for quantitative evaluations they carried out an extensive literature review involving some 500 papers. Only seven papers met the preliminary requirements for further analysis and just one survived this further stage. They concluded that while there may be data relating to the effectiveness of inter-professional education, methodological concerns, for example, about study design, lack of controls or data analysis, are at such a significant level that judgements cannot yet be made.

RELATING EDUCATION TO HEALTH CARE NEEDS

It is crucial to relate educational activities to health care needs. Four examples follow with each demonstrating a different approach. The first example, from Sweden, describes a 'training ward' for undergraduate students in the Faculty of Health Sciences at Linköping University. Here senior students from each of the health care professions rotate through two-week blocks involving day-to-day care for patients after hip replacement operations. The second example is from North America and describes a pilot project where students volunteered to work together in multiprofessional groups caring for patients with cancer. The third example is from the United Kingdom, and describes the use of a model from social psychology as the framework for a course for medical and nursing students. A further development of the model as part of the curriculum planning for a foundation course in team-work in the NHS makes up the final case description.

The 'training ward'

We have seen earlier in this book that the Faculty of Health Sciences at the University of Linköping in Sweden adopts a very broad approach to undergraduate teaching in health care. For the first 10 weeks of their first term, students from each of six health professions learn together in problem-based small groups. These students are drawn from medicine, nursing, physiotherapy, occupational therapy, bio-medical technicians and social welfare. During the 'Man and Society' element of this introduction they study aspects of ethics, health and the conditions of life. Elements of integration are then found in later parts of the course and in Term 4 the medical, nursing and physiotherapy students work together on a case study based on ischaemic heart disease. There are, in addition, shared study days on ethics, on cardiopulmonary resuscitation, and a whole week devoted to disaster medicine. These shared activities provide a firm grounding in knowledge common to each group but are not seen as effective in helping students to understand each other's roles and professional tasks (Wahlstrom et al. 1997). This awareness prompted curriculum planners to develop a series of two-week attachments to wards and practices in the area in a block called 'Team work-professional role'. The attachments were well received by students but proved very difficult to organise and administer. It was during a meeting between tutors and students that the idea of bringing students together near the end of their studies to work together on real clinical problems was raised. A central clinical facility was sought to provide a continuous experience into which students could be fitted as their timetables allowed. A small orthopaedic ward was chosen and the programme focuses predominantly on very elderly patients with hip fractures in recognition of the multiprofessional nature of the clinical and rehabilitative care required by the condition. A wide range of co-existing morbidity is also managed as part of the daily routine. The unit consists of eight beds and three teams of between six and eight students caring for patients with a variety of conditions using a three-shift rota. Rehabilitation is the central clinical focus and effective care requires efforts on both medical and social fronts. The students are responsible for all aspects of patient care from basic hygiene and medical care to clinical management and discharge arrangements. They talk to relatives, arrange social care, manage emergencies, and pre- and post-operative care. Daily ward rounds and shift handover meetings ensure continuity. There are permanent medical and nursing staff providing clinical back-up and overnight care supported by physiotherapy and occupational therapy staff. Students report considerable satisfaction with the attachments but many feel that two weeks is too short a period in which to address many of the issues raised by working together. For some it is their first opportunity to work closely with patients but all appreciate the high levels of responsibility the attachment gives them. They become aware of the skills and knowledge of their colleagues and have opportunities in regular educational sessions to discuss aspects of their professional roles and personal feelings about clinical work.

The Linköping experience reflects the first three stages of the model of learning discussed in Chapter 5 and provides students with a structured experience of progressive exposure to many of the issues involved in clinical team-working. Students are able to explore aspects of inter-professional working at a very early stage of their career in the first semester of shared group work and then have a variety of skills-building activities in later years. This final year attachment to the training ward provides a high degree of independence although for many students the principal context of their learning remains focused on their own professional skills. The short duration of the attachment and the intensity of the clinical and caring activities make the formation of a team identity difficult to achieve. Team learning occurs over issues such as ward planning, distribution of responsibilities and tasks, and roles and skills but there are few opportunities for the team to consider its strengths and weaknesses as a functional group and to begin to address these as a group.

Long-term effects of shared learning based on clinical experience

Itano and colleagues from Hawaii (1991) reported the experience of 31 students (27 female) from nursing, 4th year medical studies and social work. The students volunteered to take part in an innovative 8-week interdisciplinary oncology team-work project. They worked in teams of three and took responsibility for organising their own objectives and working methods as they developed care plans for patients with cancer and their families. The student teams took responsibility for six to eight patients with cancer over the 8-week project. They developed a care plan for each patient, attended weekly patient planning conferences, team development meetings and sessions with the clinical superviser. Other learning activities included lectures, case presentations, ward rounds, and pathological conferences. A distinctive feature of the students in this study was their maturity. The nurses were experienced registered nurses returning for a degree course, and the social work students were taking a Master's degree in social work. The medical students were in their fourth year of a typical US graduate entry medical course. To what extent this accumulated life experience contributed to the evident longer-term success of the project for these students is not clear. Certainly UK medical and nursing schools would have difficulty matching this maturity at undergraduate level and this raises important questions about relevance and timing of shared interdisciplinary learning. The example from the University of Linköping provides another innovative approach focusing on undergraduate students.

The project was successful in helping students gain team-work skills and in introducing awareness of factors influencing effective team function in a multiprofessional setting. Students were able to appreciate the need for collaboration between health care professionals when working to provide comprehensive care for patients with chronic disease. Students from the nursing and medical professions experienced considerable frustration during the project because of their difficulties in engaging with the many psycho-social elements of care they encountered. Both sets of students were aware of the various issues involved from their own training but were focused on disease management and the practical skills of physical care leaving little time for dealing with other albeit important elements of care.

Bringing professionals together: the 'contact hypothesis'

Carpenter (1995) has described a model upon which planning and evaluation of shared learning can be based. Using the 'contact hypothesis' as his starting point, Carpenter describes the planning and implementation of a course for final-year medical students and fourth-year undergraduate nursing students. The course encouraged working together in pairs and small groups on shared tasks in an atmosphere of mutual cooperation. Topics discussed included doctor–patient–nurse communications, ethical issues and deliberate self-harm among patients. Some 39 students took part in the course and reported overall improvement in attitude toward the other profession, and importantly, increased understanding of the knowledge, skills, roles and duties of the other profession. The contact hypothesis is important in this setting because it identifies those conditions that are important for success in changing attitudes when two conflicting professional groups are brought together. These factors include institutional support, a concern for the differences as well as the similarities between groups, an experience of working together as equals and the perception of each member of the group being 'typical' rather than exceptions to the perceived view of the group.

A 'foundation' course for final-year students

Parsell and her colleagues have used the principles of the contact hypothesis and combined them with other adult learning concepts to design a series of one-day 'foundation' courses for final-year students in a faculty of medicine (Parsell *et al.* 1998). In this course, students from seven professions (the professions allied to medicine [Occupational Therapy, Orthoptics, Therapy Radiography, Physiotherapy], nursing, dentistry and medicine) work in small groups on tasks related to working together in the health service. The day is focused on the transition from student to health care professional and as well as addressing issues such as the organisation of the NHS, a balance of didactic and clinical problem-solving tasks in small groups helps students identify issues concerning team-working and collaboration in the NHS. The course is very favourably reported by students, and results in improved understanding about fellow professionals and a more positive attitude towards the importance of multiprofessional team-work and communication.

NATURE OF TEAM-WORK IN PRIMARY CARE

In arguing that team-work is important in providing effective health we have assumed that there is evidence from practice that this is so. The World Health Organisation (WHO 1984, p.13) has defined the health team as:

> A group who share a common health goal and common objectives, determined by community needs, to the achievement of which each member of the team contributes, in accordance with his or her competence and skill and in co-ordination with the functions of others.

West and Poulton (1997) have explored the character of team-working in primary care in the United Kingdom. They compared 68 primary care teams with other multi-disciplinary teams using a questionnaire, the Team Climate Inventory. The questionnaire measured four aspects of team function: participation, shared objectives, task orientation and support for innovation. The comparisons were made with teams from the oil industry, social services, community mental health and NHS management. The primary care teams included general practitioners, health visitors, district nurses, practice nurses, receptionists, practice managers and other attached staff (for example, midwives, community psychiatric nurses or counsellors). The sample was broadly representative of the range of practice populations (for example, from single-handed practice to large multipartner fundholders). The average size of the primary health care teams in the sample was 18 (range 7–37). This large size was seen as more akin to 'small organisations' rather than 'teams' and the authors considered that at least some of the difficulties identified by the study could be explained by this size effect (they suggested 8–12 as the optimal size for effective teams). The study found that teams from primary health care scored significantly lower than the other teams on all team function factors except task orientation. These differences were particularly evident on the dimension relating to developing shared objectives.

A POSSIBLE FUTURE LEARNING AGENDA

In a clinical world that is undergoing what appears to be constant change, keeping up to date and responding to new initiatives are vital activities for effective health care delivery. There is a need to recognise within health care teams that there are two simultaneous agendas for learning. Not only does the team have needs regarding the development and maintenance of effective function that will include audit, performance review and task analysis, but the individual members of the team also have responsibilities for maintaining their own professional skills and knowledge. Much of these needs are pursued in professional groupings or in an *ad hoc* and solitary fashion resulting in learning alone rather than learning together. It is logical then to propose that there is a need for a *team-based* approach to continuing professional development that recognises the dual learning responsibilities of team membership. This will necessitate intra-team accountability for professional competence and growth that should stand in parallel to accountability to professional bodies and the like. Such team-based learning contracts may form part of the shared objectives of a group and be a central component of any business or development plans. Engel (1994) has classified the competencies required for effective collaboration in team-work (Table 7.1). The ideas in Table 7.1 may act as a pointer towards some of the substance of the shared learning agenda of the future, particularly where team function and growth is required.

Table 7.1 *Some competencies required for collaboration in teams (Engel 1994)*

Superordinate	Subordinate
Adapting to change	Coping with ambiguity and uncertainty Critical reasoning
Participating in change	Continuing own education
Managing self and managing others	Identifying and analysing problems, selecting appropriate means towards their resolution, monitoring progress, evaluating outcomes
Communication	Practising empathy

The separatist nature of conventional undergraduate education, so typical of undergraduate medical education but also applying to that of nurses and others, does little to foster the appropriate attitudes or awareness necessary for shared learning. Parsell and her colleagues in Liverpool (Parsell *et al.* 1998) have made some progress towards identifying what they call 'readiness' for shared learning. They have developed a short questionnaire that is based on the assumption that a student's preparedness for learning in a mixed professional grouping is related to both his or her attitudes towards their own profession and their confidence in their own role within the profession, and their awareness of the roles or responsibilities of others. The questionnaire helps students and teachers open discussion about these characteristics and to compare individuals against norms. It should prove useful in the early stages of shared educational activities and in explaining differences in response to such activities.

CONCLUSION

West and Poulton declare that 'it is clear from a wealth of previous research that teamwork is precisely the means by which the effective delivery of primary care to local populations can best be achieved' (West and Poulton 1997, p.215). We have seen from a variety of examples that there is a range of ways of setting up and running educational activities aimed at improving the awareness of participants of the knowledge and skills of the professions with whom they are going to work in the future as clinical professionals. We have also suggested that one principal aim of inter-professional education is to ensure that team-working skills are effectively introduced. Barriers to the development of an environment that will support and foster such education include institutional and political antipathy towards collaboration and change. Because collaboration does not have, of itself, any properties of spontaneous growth, it is essential that organisational support is available to encourage those who champion it (Shaw 1994). In the real world, organisations, especially those associated with the professions, strive to maintain hard-won autonomy. It will, therefore, be interesting to see the long-term outcomes of the educational experiment at Linköping. The very early introduction of shared learning into the curriculum of all the health care professions could positively influence the development of the minds and attitudes of the teachers and managers of the new century (Areskog 1988, p.252). While there is still a need for further evaluation and descriptions of good educational practice, it is becoming clearer that the days of the large group and the lecture as the main vehicles of inter-professional teaching are numbered. Small task-based and problem-based groups, using as far as possible real clinical settings and responsibilities, are emerging as the learning methods preferred by students. The use of models developed in organisational and social psychology and in human resource management to inform curriculum design brings a new dimension to the educational process. More work is necessary to develop the use of these ideas and to construct theoretical approaches to the design of educational activities that make best use of the opportunities presented by groups with often strongly held perceptions of themselves and others. The issues of 'what is a team?' and 'what is the best size for a team?' are important when considering the design of teaching materials and evaluating the effects of teaching and of learning. We have also suggested that not only should inter-professional education look at what individuals can gain from education but also that it should consider the needs of the health care team itself. The idea of 'team-based' learning encompasses concerns about accountability, flexibility and adaptability to change and the recognition that much learning in teams actually takes place outside the team within uni-professional boundaries. How much sharing of such learning subsequently takes place and how receptive other team members are to the information involved is not clear.

8

Inter-agency working

A central message of the earlier discussion has been the complexity involved in ideas about communities which are conceived in diverse ways and come in a wide variety of shapes and sizes. Community-based practice, and by extension, professional education for such practice, have to recognise that complexity and prepare staff to cope effectively with the challenges and opportunities which it presents. Those challenges and opportunities were very evident in Chapter 7 which discussed the extended network of professions working within the various communities and the educational needs generated in preparing professionals who can network more effectively. This chapter deals with another aspect of that networking. As we saw, inter-professional work is difficult in itself, but is made more difficult by the fact that the professions involved work within a range of organisations which display wide variations in their structure, culture and function. The significance of these varied contexts for the way in which professionals work, and the constraints and opportunities generated by the varied organisations, are important issues which figure much less in current professional education than the rhetoric about multi-disciplinary practice might suggest.

Approaching these issues from an organisational perspective reminds us that much of the professional context is determined by the many non-professional players working within most organisations and often having significant effect on their operation. This introduces issues onto the agenda which extend the narrow traditional focus of professional concern and accept the complexity both of communities and of organisations within them. Many doctors have been trained within the established context of hospital organisation but many have struggled with the changes being experienced in those relatively closed organisations. The more open structure of many community-based organisations adds significant complicating factors for those playing professional roles within them. This gives the issue special significance in relation to community-based practice though it should be observed that any enhanced organisational awareness which results would also be useful for those destined to work in more conventional hospital settings.

This extension of professional concerns to include aspects of organisations has another characteristic in that it naturally extends into consideration of the relevance of organisations to the more extended roles which community-based professionals might play. The earlier discussion about settings for community learning concentrated on them being suitable sites which could provide alternative learning opportunities for the development of the traditional skills practised within health care. It is argued that patients may as well be seen within a community-based health centre or in an individual doctor's surgery as in an out-patient clinic or on a hospital ward. That conception of the purpose of community settings might be extended to include seeing people, though not of course as patients, within the confines of a social agency or voluntary project. The significance of experience in these diverse community settings, however, goes beyond patient contact even in those with a narrowly medical focus. They offer the professional in training an opportunity to experience the impact of the setting, and of the organisational context, on core professional practice and on the more extended definition of the professional role. Maximisation of the benefits of such experiences requires a much greater emphasis on relevant subjects in the content of early education, and in the choice of placements which can highlight issues of organisation and context in relation to professional practice. Long-standing efforts among community-based doctors in the United Kingdom to retain their independent contractor status in relation to the health service, and evidence of problems between partners where they have come together in quite simple organisations, confirm the importance of this approach to organisational experience.

The diversity of relevant agencies in the community becomes more significant when they are seen not only as a locus for patient contact, but also as having relevance for health conditions within the area, and for the more complex treatment and prevention of those conditions. Here it is not so much a question of experiencing practice within another agency, but more a matter of understanding agencies, what they provide, how they operate and the constraints under which they work. This is relevant at the level of individual patient care, where the referral capacity within, for example, the GP role as provider of comprehensive and coordinated care, depends on such knowledge. It is also relevant where that role is extended, as in the latest proposals in the United Kingdom, to consider the health concerns of the practice population, or of a much wider population in relation to commissioning for their hospital care (Secretary of State 1997). This is extended further when the professional role in developing better health is considered more broadly and extends to joint action for health, or where professional advocacy is directed at changing the policy and practice of other agencies.

CHARACTERISTICS OF ORGANISATIONS

Chapter 4 outlined the complex agency and organisational structure present in communities and varying with the approach taken to the definition of community. There was no singular concept of community which would serve all purposes and the varied levels at which community might be conceived inter-relate in complicated ways. The resulting patterns of mutual influence across the boundaries between communities are as complicated and as significant as those across the boundaries between the sectors and the professions involved within, and related to, health and health care. Such complexity does not lend itself easily to approaches which involve the direct, experiential learning which dominates traditional health care education. It is not simply a matter of experience in one or two relevant organisations. As with the core content of clinical education for health care, there is a common basis which underlies the study of organisations and which provides the foundations for the later more detailed development of skills and capacities in relation to particular roles in particular organisations. Factors which are common to organisations will be emphasised in such an approach and the relevance of key organisational characteristics will also become apparent. Transferability of skills and experience between organisations will then be easier and the appropriateness of diverse community experience takes on added significance. With this emphasis the selection of pivotal organisations where students may learn will rest as much on their value in exemplifying such key organisational characteristics as on their capacity to provide salient clinical opportunities (Wasylenki *et al.* 1997).

This process of understanding the generic features of organisations involves drawing on literature which falls outside the mainstream of professional medical education. If the community perspective is to become more important and if effective practice in the community is to be developed, it needs to be seen as a part of the core, perhaps for all, but certainly for those intending to enter community-based practice.

WHY ARE ORGANISATIONS IMPORTANT?

In an era of change and one in which economy and accountability are becoming more significant as criteria by which health services are judged, it is important to be clear about the significance of organisations. Historical evidence about institutional change within health care confirms the significance which professionals attach to the context within which they work, and illustrates their capacity to maintain both the organisational structures and their relationship with them, over long periods of time (Klein 1989). This reflects their awareness of the importance of such factors and their traditional ability to influence organisation to facilitate their own practice. Their ability to deal with more radical change is much more in doubt. This has been increasingly evident as the momentum of health care reform has gathered pace and as the dynamics of the change process have led to reforms being imposed on, rather than negotiated with, the medical profession, or at least being perceived in that way (Boaden 1997). Such reforms have perhaps tended to increase the division between professional practice and organisational intentions so that professional education which assumes established positions of power and influence in relation to stable organisations may become less productive in an era of rapid organisational change.

Resources lie at the heart of the changing climate in which organisations and professionals are operating. As was shown in Chapter 1, developed countries are showing increased concern about the levels of public spending involved in health care and considerations of economy and efficiency are increasingly being raised with service delivery organisations. Resource constraints imposed by government may require substantial organisational change, and even with such change, seem likely to have direct impact on service provision and so on the style and content of professional work. Rationing of health care is the most visible manifestation of this with the front-line professionals often being the visible instrument of rationing because of remote and unseen changes in resource flows (Harrison and Hunter 1994). Provision of resources to organisations is a complicated matter. It depends on the character of the health care system, as was seen earlier, but also on the formal structures developed for the delivery of care. Allocation to the organisation is of course only the first level of concern with detailed control of resource allocation within organisations varying widely. Decisions about the more detailed use of resources at the point of service delivery also vary but this has been the point at which professional autonomy has been seen as of paramount importance. General limitations on overall resourcing have changed the context for that autonomy significantly and in the United Kingdom there is some evidence of direct controls over clinical behaviour being dictated by resource constraint (Boaden 1997).

Recent evidence in the United Kingdom about the struggles over budgets within health care illustrates the issues very clearly. Political and financial managers are clearly accountable for the use of public resources but must exercise their control of spending through the professional staff who are best able to determine the detailed pattern of resource use and are in many cases the real resource. Control of that end use becomes most important in such a context if the gap between policy intentions determined within management hierarchies and implementation in practice is to be minimised. Efforts to manage these relationships are complicated within organisations, and attempts to manage compliance and establish congruence between organisations through the introduction of market mechanisms into inter-agency relations has not proved always straightforward in the health field (Le Grand and Bartlett 1993).

This issue is compounded in the community where the potential range of organisations with useful resources which may be applied to health and health care is so much wider. Referral may be the chosen method by which professionals access the resources of other professions and organisations, but it is the decisions of those to whom referrals are made which will determine successful access and the quality of subsequent care (Ovretveit 1993). This is evident in the response when referrals are perceived as inappropriate by the receivers, and the implications when care cannot be regulated at the point of access are evident in the impact of discharges into the community where the resource implications may be less controllable because of the character of community care. This has always been problematic within the community where many referrals are outside the clinical arena where doctors' knowledge and understanding of the work of other professions have not been good, and where understanding of the constraints under which other professions operate has been largely missing.

These issues are clearly relevant in treating individual cases, but they assume greater significance when seen in the aggregate, although that is seldom done. Individual professionals learn ways of gaining access for their patients or clients and seek successful ways of engaging existing systems. The argument for changes in those systems is, as a result, often not presented and the implications of this for patients in general may be significant. Practitioners vary in their capacity and willingness to 'play the game' in relation to their patients, and all practitioners learn the limits of the existing systems. In recognising the need not to overburden systems they limit their own demands (hidden rationing) and systems are not alerted to the need to change their own resource allocations because demand remains latent. Current concerns about Accident and Emergency Units in the United Kingdom epitomise the problem with traditional behaviour by professionals and patients creating excessive demands (Williams *et al.* 1997). This is not a new phenomenon, but has been exacerbated in its impact by resource constraints within both sectors of care, changes in hospital and primary care practice, and the development of an internal market which has had severe consequences for the management of both primary and secondary care. The result has been crisis management of a chronic situation which has built up over many years as a result of developed practices in some areas of primary care, and learned patient behaviour in relation to medical services. Dealing with one's own situational problems at the expense of other parts of an integrated health care system is not necessarily the best way to proceed. Alternative strategies of course rely on much more knowledge about the wider system and how its constituent parts work.

This analysis may be extended to cover a much wider range of concerns but there is no need to do so in order to establish the point. Rather, it is necessary to establish the features of agencies and organisations which may be relevant to both an understanding of organisations and to the development of the skills needed in order to exploit that greater understanding.

WHAT ARE THE KEY FEATURES OF ORGANISATIONS?

The broad classification of community organisations outlined earlier offered an initial view of a number of key dimensions of organisations which might be relevant to health care professionals and educators. Here we want to examine organisations in more detail to develop that typology in ways which would equip professional students for their core roles within community-based health care, and deal with those extensions of role which develop with experience.

The extensive list of relevant organisations within the community is testimony to a number of important factors which are relevant. An understanding of aim and purpose may be put first, partly because it is relatively straightforward. It is especially relevant in community-based health care as the range of relevant organisations is widened greatly by this emphasis. It is clear within the context of treatment that patients are often treated by staff working in a wide range of organisations, and that specialisation has produced a narrowing of the focus of interest of each organisation. Some agencies of course are invested with overall responsibility for a range of such specialties and face complex organisation challenges in managing that range.

THE GEOGRAPHY OF ORGANISATIONS

It has been stressed repeatedly that community is a complex idea and it is important for our purposes to recognise the multi-layered notion of community. In the absence of any clear geographical definition then communities must be considered at a number of scalar levels which will coincide with variable patterns of public interaction, but importantly from our perspective, will relate to clear organisational structures. Table 8.1 represents this idea illustrating the levels with examples drawn from health care. In terms of services the highly specialised teaching hospital serves a large population and a wider 'community' than the District General Hospital, while the Polyclinic serves a wider population than does the group practice or the solo general practitioner. Indeed, the latter do not serve a catchment population, but their registered patients, which means that the smaller local community may be highly fragmented for these purposes. This is an important example in relation to health care in so far as patients are referred across the community boundaries of each level for various aspects of their health care treatment. There is much discussion about the appropriateness of these structures in relation to people's sense of identity and the argument for the very local catchment of UK general practice has depended largely on local identity and accessibility. Use of A and E departments, however, suggests a willingness among patients to self-refer quite long distances for diagnosis and treatment where their experience suggests that their local practitioner would refer them in any case, or that it is an equally accessible and acceptable way to secure immediate treatment.

This obvious division within health care is important for these reasons but also because the different scales of operation greatly influence the way in which health care delivery is organised and the context within which professionals must operate in their community-based practice. This becomes significantly more complex if one adds to the map those organisations who have command over the resourcing and accountability of health care provision and the many other types of agency and organisation who may have a bearing on the health and health care of populations. This is done in Table 8.2.

It is immediately evident that there are large numbers of organisations at each level of community and that their inter-relationship is significant to the delivery of effective and equitable care. If the developing professional is to engage with this complexity, there is a need for education and training to equip them for dealing with

Table 8.1 *Scale of service delivery in relation to direct health care services*

Scale of service	Organisation
Region	Teaching Hospital
District	District General Hospital Community Trust Health Authority
Locality	Large Health Centre Polyclinic Commissioning Group
Sub-Locality	Small General Practice Devolved Outreach facility Community Pharmacist

Table 8.2 *Scale of service delivery in relation to health and related services*

Scale of service	Health care services	Related services
Region	Teaching Hospital	
District	District General Hospital Health Authority Community Trust	Social Services Department Local Education Authority Local Housing Department
Locality	Polyclinic Large Health Centre Commissioning Group	Social Services District Office
Sub-Locality	Small General Practice Devolved Outreach facility Community Pharmacist	Local School Local Housing Office Detached Youth or Drug Workers Housing Association Neighbourhood Association

complex relationships and not merely with other professional staff. It is one of the remarkable things about recent years that the case conference as a part of the care process, and the occasional public enquiry when that process goes radically wrong, have become part of the fabric of health and social care delivery. Both tend to focus on the need for inter-professional work, but the latter highlight issues of resource constraint, lack of training, poor management, supervision and communication which are often as much about organisational failure as they are about inadequate professional practice. This makes it more surprising that so little attention is devoted to the dynamics of organisations and of inter-organisational relationships in the training of participant staff.

Much greater clarity about the nature of organisations and the dynamics of their operation and decision-making are needed for sensitive inter-agency activity to take place. The model which saw referral as moving responsibility for the patient to another professional or organisation is not appropriate to the complex budgets of agencies and the difficulty in apportioning responsibility for care, and the interactive character of much care as patients move between sectors and between specialties. If community-based practice involves moving beyond the concern with individual patients to examine the health of whole populations, then the need for understanding of the wider organisational network becomes even more pronounced.

It is at this second stage that what needs to be understood is greatly extended. In fact there is an argument for suggesting that in relation to individual cases, personal advocacy may be more successful. Certainly, knowledge about organisational constraints and tight organisational policies controlling professional action may greatly inhibit compliance in that kind of interaction. The alternative is for professionals to engage in a wider advocacy which is concerned to shift such policy guidelines so that individual advocacy is less significant and normal action more acceptable. This may involve resource questions but that is what is required, rather than an avoidance of those questions by a reversion to dealing with individual cases, and the unequal outcomes that traditionally characterise that process.

What, then, may be said about organisations once they have been mapped onto the geographical area in this way? There are a number of characteristics which are important and which condition the actions of organisations and about which professionals need to know both while training and when engaged in practice. These include the aims and purposes of the organisation, the character of its personnel and its formal structure and informal practices, the distribution of power and influence within an organisation, the source of resource for an organisation, the form of accountability, and so forth. These all deserve some treatment here although this is not a text book on organisations.

ORGANISATIONAL AIMS

This is an aspect of organisations and agencies which becomes of much greater significance when health care professionals move into the community. Even within health care, organisations have a different character from hospitals and are exposed to the much broader and more random impact of public demand for services. The fact that most of these services provide first contact care imposes additional burdens on them which are removed from hospitals which are screened, in the main, from such direct demand. The problems at A and E epitomise this distinction within the hospital sector and have their greatest impact when their consequences impact on the capacity of the acute care service delivery.

Within the community the presence of unexpected issues and the wider orientation to their treatment present problems for organisations. On the one hand, it is possible, and indeed has been a strong traditional model, to see them as analogous to hospitals, simply there to provide treatment in a community setting. The nature of treatment differs in so far as they have a responsibility to refer where more complex treatment may be needed, and much of the treatment delivered directly is of a limited kind. That narrow view is greatly extended if one takes into account the issues of health promotion and disease prevention which arise in the community setting, as well as the provision of support, care and advice which are not essentially clinical, but fall by convention and practice within the health care arena.

The point here is that such extensions of aim pose challenges to organisations, partly because they involve change in the initial stages, and partly because these added objectives may require different forms of organisation and practice, different resource allocations and perhaps the use of different professional staff. The history of reform has been one in which these extensions of function have been introduced without reference to such factors and organisations with a quite different programme of aims have been expected to adopt the new tasks, and presumably adapt to their provision. Sometimes resources have been provided to cope with the change, sometimes not.

This is a relatively straightforward point well understood by most professionals within organisations when the organisation requires them to undertake extended functions which they often resist in the name of professional autonomy or quality standards. It is that very resistance, and the need within organisations to manage greater compliance, which make the character of organisation so important. Understanding organisational structures and the dynamics of decision-making are important, both to those who wish to maintain their traditional autonomy and to those who wish to comply, or secure wider compliance.

This is even more the case when inter-agency exchanges are demanded by a situation whether in relation to direct patient care, or in the wider context of disease prevention or health promotion. The organisations involved beyond those within health care have their own sets of aims, objectives and purposes and they create the context in which referrals or other approaches will be received. A referral is no more than an invitation to another professional or agency to examine a case and determine whether, and if so, what they may do with that referral. Custom and practice may have normalised some referral patterns but there is increasing concern to establish more codified ways of handling such relationships and often the motivation for such developments lies within core features of the organisations involved. Some of these relate to purpose, and the possibility that inappropriate referrals may well deflect activity outside the normal remit, or change the composition of work so that the organisation is no longer determining its own programmes. This again is a long-standing feature of many inter-organisational and indeed inter-professional relationships and has been dealt with often through individual decisions by agency staff, and by learned sensitivities in relation to inter-agency relationships. Once issues move beyond that level there is greater need for clarity about organisational factors and the possibility of altering the context within which professional and other staff are taking decisions.

ORGANISATIONAL STRUCTURES

Clearly, aim and purpose set important parameters to organisational activity, but in terms of inter-agency relationships, the dynamics are more influenced by other factors which may derive from such aims. Organisations are usually established with explicit purposes in mind and structured to deliver those main purposes. There are a variety of typologies of organisation which relate to the issue of prime purpose and these may be illustrated in relation to community health and related organisations. This can be seen, for example, in relation to the development of minor surgery within general practice, or the extension of health visitor services to deal with the elderly as well as dealing with children. In both cases the tasks involved fall broadly within the professional training of the doctors and health visitors involved, but the organisational dynamics are quite different. In minor surgery the timing of treatment and the equipment and staffing necessary to its conduct are different from the conventional models of general practice consultations. In addition the skills involved may have once been learned, but are different from those conventionally exercised within general practice. The result may be a degree of specialisation within a generalist model and the consequent need for a larger group of doctors to work together to allow some to develop that specialist capability. In relation to both work content, measures of workload and performance criteria, there may be a need to extend organisational judgements and accept more diverse colleague activity.

In the health visitor case the issue is different. The long-established concern with children is exercised within a system of ante-natal care, child delivery within a medical context and registration and statutory requirements dictating involvement. The organisational requirements to meet this task are not simple but they are clear-cut and supported by these features of the clientele. The case of the elderly is different. In the absence of demand, and that might be mediated through other agencies or informal carers, organisations need to be pro-active in seeking to provide support. This in itself is complicated, and support is made more difficult because the range of concerns and appropriate interventions falls well outside the direct capacities of the health visitors involved. The need for financial advice and the difficult transitions involved in housing decisions for the elderly loom large but have to be dealt with by other agencies. Carers often need support and sometimes respite which again are services provided elsewhere than within health visiting. There are of course invaluable services which health visitors can provide, but there is a risk that that will dictate the patterns of intervention and support, unless organisations take on board the wider purpose. Then there will need to be a heightened capacity to act in inter-agency ways in order that they may act as gatekeepers to needed services.

So what features of organisation might be relevant to the delivery of such changed functions, and relevant by extension to many other organisational developments and interactions within the community? Prominent among them might be organisational size. The archetypal model of individualised professional practice has become increasingly rare among those who once practised in that way, and for many health professions has never formally applied to their work. The community-based physician best epitomises that tradition but single-handed practice is in decline, and the pressures to develop larger group practice, wider groupings of doctors and associated staff, and even larger groupings for other purposes are now very evident. In such cases organisation comes into play. Situationally in relation to individual cases it may be possible to operate idiosyncratically and autonomously, but collective activity challenges that mode. Patients may not see the same practitioner, or even a doctor, on each visit, and they may as a result come to expect more uniform processes and standards of care from whoever they see. This may be reinforced by the fact that the larger organisation, especially where it is publicly funded, has to account for its use of resources and defend variation in its practice in a way which was less apparent when practice was fragmented. This requires organisation.

One corollary of greater size is often the need for devolved practice within the organisation. In terms of our geographical mapping (see Table 8.1) the organisation appears in sector two or even three because of the formal range of population involved and the numbers of staff needed. Best direct practice, however, may be better engaged within sector one where the population is more accessible and where a shared sense of local identification may be important. Such devolved practice may encourage and facilitate autonomy on the part of professional staff, and if the organisation wishes to exercise controls this may necessitate much higher levels of record keeping and reporting than was traditionally the case. This has been evident with the advent of fundholding and other market-driven changes where resourcing has changed and with that change has gone a need for much closer scrutiny of spending to secure accountability. This has been an object of much criticism by professionals, many of whom resent the intrusion on their autonomy, but the alternative traditional model would imply that the financial implications of clinical decision-making are no different to the clinical decisions themselves, which is clearly not the case. The rationale for accountability derives from that difference and organisations increasingly need to engage with such controls and professional staff to maintain recording which permits that to occur. Failure to do so means that a key element of accountability is lost, as was often the case historically when little was known about how resources were used, or to what effect. This has become even more important with the emergence of performance criteria, comparative evaluation of staff and organisations and payment by results in relation to some aspects of health care.

These considerations lead into well-rehearsed issues around organisations concerning their degree of formalisation, a characteristic often absent from traditional models of community-based health care. It is ironic that in many cases of more conventional organisation high degrees of formalisation are associated with large-scale productivity and a degree of routinisation in the work. This has always been regarded as the antithesis of professional practice where the individualistic features of cases have been argued as the justification for looseness of structure and specification. Ironically in much community-based practice, the scale of activity is very high and the character of much of the work is relatively routine. This would seem to be an ideal scenario for formalisation of activity and the establishment of routines for the exercise of work. This itself is present in the criteria developed over patients' rights in the UK NHS which specify appointment times and waiting times for treatment or consultation as basic aspects of patients' rights. These are the stuff of routine administrative systems and belie the fact that the skills being exercised in the consultation are argued to be highly developed, demand autonomy for their exercise and should not be under the control of anyone other than professional staff. The clear conflict between the criteria, and the imperatives they present to organisations illustrate the pressures under which professionals now work, pressures which are causing a rethink about the organisation of some professional work and the division of labour which should operate where the skill mix within the case load is incongruent with the skill mix of the individual professions (Jenkins-Clarke *et al.* 1997).

This leads naturally into consideration of a further aspect related to size though not always present in large organisations, namely the complexity of the organisation. The archetypal professional organisation used to be very simple, involving one professional, or a small number, operating with modest support staff of a non-professional kind. Increases in scale have changed this model and now it is common to find several professions working together within the same organisation leading to divisions of labour, and often of associated organisation, which are difficult to prescribe. Boundaries become critical to the work of the organisation. If they are very clear, they may inhibit the extension of proper professional concern in relation to cases. If they are blurred, there may be extensive disputes about staff working beyond the proper boundaries of their professional competence. These are issues for all organisation but there may be added problems when responsibility for care and for expenditure is being apportioned, because unclear boundaries make that more difficult to do.

ORGANISATIONAL PROCESSES

These issues of structure are the visible aspects of organisation and are usually enshrined in the formal arrangements. In no organisation do they prescribe all the operational practices, however, in most cases merely providing a framework against which informal patterns of working relationship can evolve, dictating some practices but leaving varied degrees of discretion to staff in relation to others. These informal patterns are the essence of most concern to all staff, but most particularly to professional staff where their formal skills are involved. The tension between the traditions of professional autonomy and the demands and constraints imposed by formal structure generate the key pressure points where issues of power, influence and authority arise. The formal structures tend to prescribe the authority patterns in any organisation and they may or may not correspond to the more complex patterns of power and influence which develop in any organisation.

In the archetypal professional practice authority, power and influence would coincide, with the professional having formal and informal control and exercising all three. Placing professionals within more complex organisations tends to lead to uncertainty about where each will be exercised. Other professions may be involved seeking at least equivalence in formal terms, while management roles may involve staff whose status is regarded as non-professional and whose impact on professional practice is often resented. Resolution of such issues may be enshrined in the formal structure adopted or it may be a matter of less formal sanctions being applied, or of influence being exercised using a variety of resources in order to achieve control over what are seen to be key aspects of performance.

These features are related to questions of decision-making and organisational leadership and to the broad area of communication within organisations. For those who think that the traditional professional model should be extended beyond the core and into more complex areas of practice, this poses problems. The complexity and accountability patterns of organisations where this is intended raise issues which are not consistent with traditional professional models. Power usually lies with formal position in the organisation, and less formal influence has to be earned through operating within the organisation. Formal authority is often invested in non-professional staff as it is, for example, in most politicised organisations where public accountability gives significant authority to lay managers and ultimate authority to elected politicians.

EDUCATIONAL IMPLICATIONS

Recognition of such factors and of their relevance and importance for practice poses sharp challenges to professionals and to those who are designing curricula and teaching courses within professional schools. There are immediate implications in terms of what students should know, how they should approach learning and how lifelong professional development should be engaged. Some of these are implicit in the earlier discussion of learning styles but there is a need for that discussion to be related more directly to these specific areas of substantive concern within broader community-based education and practice. As with clinical skills, so in relation to community-based organisations, it is a matter of where, when and how, knowledge, understanding and organisational skills may best be learned.

The intellectual basis for understanding organisations involves a range of disciplines which fall outside the conventional medical curriculum, or when they fall within it, are being engaged with an entirely different focus. So, for example, medical students will engage with some psychology and sociology, but always in the context of a patient-oriented approach to their own professional practice. Both subjects have relevance for the study of organisations, but are usually treated differently in order to focus on the specific concerns of the traditional core professional task. So too have a number of other disciplines, not least the formal study of organisations, itself now established as an independent discipline, often associated with formal study of management. To these may be added a number of areas of study of political science, systems analysis and soft systems methodology, all of which have been applied to the analysis and understanding of organisational behaviour.

Clearly, these are not central to the core of professional practice unless perhaps doctors go on to specialise in public health where their relevance is much more obviously apparent. In other cases they become significant, and for some they become core concerns in relation to areas of practice which emerge in later medical careers and often prove problematic for practitioners when they do arise. The absence of a grounding in relevant disciplines creates problems which are not easily overcome in a continuing professional context where much education and further training has to be engaged with limited time available and within the ongoing work setting. The experiential opportunities are then constrained by such practicalities often imposed by the very constraints that such education and training is seeking to manage or remove.

Providing for this combination of base knowledge and experiential opportunity poses a serious challenge to those organising preparation for placements in the community. The intellectual foundations necessary for good experiential opportunities necessarily involve learning some of the basic outlines of disciplines not currently within the normal curriculum. These will require teaching, almost always, by specialists who fall outside the staff of the medical school. Such staff will need to develop a knowledge of health services and their organisation in order to illustrate their teaching and student learning with appropriate material which has relevance and of course relates to the subsequent experiences which students may have in the community. This is important, as we have seen, because the character of organisations varies and so much of the current material about organisations derives from sources within the commercial and business fields. While such examples have relevance, their particular characteristics may be less appropriate and their ethos may be very different and so misleading.

The organisation of community placements is equally difficult. Given the range of possibilities it is clear that attachments need to be sensitively organised to match the stage of student development and the particular learning needs evident at different stages in that development. For example, students may be developing clinical capacities which allow them to prioritise their treatment activity, but this needs to be seen within its organisational setting. This may involve, for example, a placement in a health authority, perhaps shadowing a manager during some part of the annual budgetary process. This would allow the student to observe the inevitable prioritising which goes on, and the key influences operating within the broader allocation process within which their own activity takes place. It would also allow them an insight into the impact of their own decisions in terms of other services offered by professional colleagues, but also on support services which underpin the range of professional activity. The management of competing demands may provide a useful framework both for the consideration of case priorities, but also for the gathering of broader evidence which may better inform the budget process.

Enough has been said to illustrate the breadth of this agenda and its complexity. It is probable that initial professional education will only provide the groundwork for development in this complex area. This will open the way for more effective continuing education but that in turn will require considerable development and forms the subject of the next chapter.

9

Continuing education for community practice

The discussion so far has concentrated largely on initial professional education and the changes which will be required there if the challenges and opportunities inherent in future community-based practice are to be met. Some reference has been made to the current postgraduate educational system which has been designed to prepare conventional medical graduates for community-based practice, but the limitations of that system, and more particularly of any continuing career-long education have been remarked. This is a situation shared by all the professions where the emphasis is placed on initial education and admission to the profession, and where the demands imposed by practice in later professional life militate against involvement in continuing education. This does not mean that continuing education is not important throughout a professional career. The current concerns in medicine with promoting evidence-based and reflective practice confirm the need for professionals to maintain and develop their knowledge and skills throughout the career. The current efforts being made in medical education to give entrants to the profession the attitudes and competencies associated with self-directed and lifelong learning acknowledge this need and that it is not being met.

The emphasis placed on this aspect of curriculum reform has been remarked throughout the text. Indeed, in many of the examples considered it has seemed more important than the issues related to the development of community-based practice itself and the substantive challenges which that presents to intending practitioners.

This emphasis is entirely consistent with the current limitations within the formal systems of continuing medical education which mean that self-direction has to be seen as a principal way forward. At the same time the approach seems to reflect an assumption that the career profiles of future doctors will continue along the well-defined and relatively conventional tracks established in the past. Self-direction within those limits currently takes place and the enhanced opportunities offered in current medical schools should enhance career-long performance. It is less likely to be adequate to meet the needs and demands placed on future health care professionals, particularly those being met within a changing and developing community-based practice.

The argument being presented here is that an essential characteristic of future health care is that it will be different from the current system, and that the system will continue to change, making flexibility and adaptability central characteristics of professional careers. Self-directed continuing education may be adequate to meet that challenge, but in doing so it will have to support innovative activity by those professionals who will lead the changes and considerable adaptive and organisational skill among those who will have to adopt the innovative ideas. Even with a heightened capacity for self-directed learning among new professionals the likely character of the future learning agenda suggests that there will be a need for much more elaborate support systems to be available to individual professionals throughout their later careers. Within professional practice there will be a need to resource the care system adequately to provide time and opportunity for continuing education. Within the education system there will be a need to provide the learning resources and the personal support systems to enable professionals to make good use of those opportunities which are made available.

Before looking at these, and other, issues in more detail it is important to remember the two distinct elements of the model of developed career practice within the community which have been discussed throughout the text so far. One is the need for professionals to maintain and develop the areas of core practice which remain within their continuing role. The boundaries of that role may change, and so may some aspects of what were core functions, but it is likely that many core activities will not change. What will change are the knowledge base and skills involved in the provision of those core functions and the attitudes of patients being cared for. What will not change, but may need greater attention in the future, is the need to develop the personal qualities that constitute a significant part of community practice both in relation to patients and their informal carers and to the members of the more complex primary health care teams which are developing.

At the same time, alongside these core roles, there will be additional new roles to be played which result from the widened perspective involved in the more developed forms of community-based practice. In time some of these may develop so far as to define a new core, while others are likely to be less universal in their practice, being played by some professionals within teams but not by others. Economic arguments will drive such changes in many cases, but there are also professional arguments for changes in the definition of roles and the blending of the varied professional skills to be found within the new teams. Certainly the creation of community-based health care teams carries with it an implicit expectation of greater specialisation.

CONTINUING EDUCATION FOR CORE PRACTICE

Continuing education to maintain and develop core practice is of course not new. There is a current expectation that professionals will maintain, up-date and develop their practice, but this is an area in which their performance in doing so is difficult to monitor and evaluate. On the one hand, there is often some disagreement about what constitutes the core of practice and there is also a very strong sense of the individuality of professional practice which makes judgement about performance very difficult. Comparative evidence about individual practice is often not accepted as valid and the establishment of agreed baseline standards is consequently difficult. In any case, agreement about criteria would not of itself solve the problem given the absence of readily available data about the activity and outcome of much community-based practice. The introduction of a system of re-accreditation as has happened in some countries would help to establish the legitimacy of periodic evaluation of performance, but the difficulty of making judgements within such a system often leads to the establishment of minimal criteria rather than developmental standards which might serve to raise average performance in the profession as a whole.

Leaving aside this difficult issue of standards, UK general practice offers an interesting case study of continuing professional education in relation to current practice. Three key elements of any such system are in place and are able to benefit from the fact that they follow a common period of professional vocational training undertaken by all those involved. The system is generously funded, certainly by comparison with the resources available to other professions working within the community. Some £50 million is spent each year in income to general practitioners which is contingent on them each attending 30 hours of continuing education. The content of that education is specified in the requirements of the system which involve clinical knowledge, health promotion and practice management as the three core areas of study. This goes some way towards recognising a broadly defined core curriculum, but it is highly general and the detail of courses or learning opportunities offered within those headings varies widely. Finally the system has now put in place a national system of GP Tutors who operate in localities to facilitate the development and take-up of continuing education by their colleagues. In addition but outside this formal system most professionals engage with other ways of up-dating and developing their professional knowledge and skills though they may not always define this as continuing education, rather seeing it as a part of their normal professional practice.

The impact of this system is difficult to determine. Evidence about practice remains elusive and consequently so does evidence about the impact of education on practice. Most evaluation is confined within the educational setting dealing with direct feedback about the educational experience and reported learning, often immediately after the learning period. The longer-term impact of education is much more difficult to evaluate and in a complex area where many factors are influencing professional behaviour it would be difficult to isolate the independent impact of continuing education. This should not limit the search for better evidence and the development of measures of effective and efficient practice and of effective education. Such output measures are often lost sight of in the dominant concern with inputs to the system of continuing education whether this relates to the character of the educational experience itself or to the decisions by doctors about which educational sessions to attend. This is similar to the concerns within initial professional training which have been discussed earlier in the text where questions about how to engage with mature professional learners heavily outweigh concern with possible changes in what they need to learn and why they should be learning.

Questions about the educational process are of course important but their domination is partly possible because most continuing education currently falls within the areas of traditional knowledge and skill which were well established in medical schools in the past. Extension of professional concerns in community-based care is likely to focus attention back on to content as well as process, and would require a debate within the profession about individual autonomy and the diversity of practice for it to be effectively considered. The result is that the system deals reasonably well with the standard elements of traditional medical up-dating including elements related to new diseases, and more often, new treatments, particularly in the field of drug use. There are also new areas of practice like minor surgery where community-based practitioners have had to re-hone skills not practised since their hospital days. These are relatively straightforward matters and are now being dealt with in the context of more aware adult educational approaches like those discussed earlier which no doubt enhance the educational experience and deepen the learning.

More difficult in the context of core development are the personal qualities associated with better and more effective practice. It is clear in what has been said earlier that much community-based practice does not involve the regular exercise of complicated clinical skills and judgement. The principle of open access adopted in community-based health care, and years of reactive practice in face of high levels of demand, mean that large numbers of people continue to present with self-limiting conditions and with minor injuries and ailments which require modest treatment which falls within the professional skill of practice nurses as well as doctors. There are of course within that large group of patients others with more severe conditions at various stages of development and there are those with chronic conditions which require treatment and support of a continuing but semi-specialist nature. Even in these cases, however, many conditions require skills that are less to do with detailed medical knowledge and more to do with interactive skills and a wide knowledge of both the sources of stress and the community resources available to assist with them. Indeed, in many cases care for the patient is coupled with increasing concern with the informal carers, family and neighbours, who support such patients for most of the time but who are often exposed to stress-induced conditions themselves as a consequence.

This agenda raises clear issues about the personal aspects of professional development which were discussed in Chapter 6. Developments such as mentoring, portfolio learning and the consequences of small group learning are beginning to create the potential for these issues to be addressed and some are being addressed more directly. One area which deals with one aspect of concern is the heavy emphasis being placed on the development of communication skills, although this is much less prevalent within continuing education when compared with vocational training for community practice. Once again it would seem that this is seen as a skill appropriate to be developed in initial training and then left to the individual to maintain and refine within his or her own practice rather than relying on a significant contribution from formal continuing education. One result is a much wider diversity of practice in this respect than might be acceptable in a community-based system where economy and equity of treatment are key criteria of performance. Concerns about consulting style are central to this concern with communication and this immediately raises the question of individual autonomy discussed earlier. At the same time it is an issue which lies at the heart of professional practice, with consulting style and the length of consultations having considerable bearing on both diagnosis and treatment. There is some evidence that practitioners adopt the consulting mode which fits their preferred type of practice, and there is wide variation, but the growth of consumerism and patient influence could perhaps change that direction to establish what best fits the patient's needs.

Despite this reservation, the current system serves some aspects of core development reasonably well. More marginal issues and those which fall outside well-established clinical guidelines are not so commonly dealt with and areas like audit, research and development remain relatively under-nourished within the established system of continuing education, being regarded as a separate activity in a compartmentalised way. What is even less well served is the development of non-core activities and of the professional's ability to engage with change within practice and in the context of practice.

CONTINUING EDUCATION FOR NON-CORE DEVELOPMENT

If the maintenance and development of core professional activity pose sharp challenges to established systems of continuing education, then the challenge posed by non-core development and innovatory practice is clearly profound. It has been argued throughout the text that these latter areas are those where the community-based health care of the future has to develop. Merely to list functions such as pro-active population-based practice, active advocacy in the wider community in relation to health promotion and prevention, research and development as a corporate concern in future community-based practice and management of, or participation in, the wider primary health care team illustrates the challenge faced by continuing education.

It could be argued that some of these concerns fall somewhere within the current undergraduate programme, but the evidence suggests that the coverage offered there is not adequate to prepare professionals for the challenges ahead. All these extensions of role pose difficult challenges for continuing education, especially when initial professional education has concentrated on core activity, and where more peripheral knowledge and skills have been dealt with only superficially and have not been used and developed systematically in early practice.

In order to address such problems continuing professional education will need a radical overhaul. The elements discussed in the case of UK general practice discussed earlier are all necessary, but they need to be oriented to the future needs of community-based care. This involves appropriate resourcing, applied not to reward the practitioner, but to enable the practice organisation to create the space and time to facilitate effective study. This in turn raises questions about the organisation and management of practice in order to facilitate continuing education, especially around what are currently more peripheral concerns. Changes in these areas would help to foster the demand side of continuing education. In turn this would need to be met by the creation of an effective supply side in order not to frustrate that expressed demand. This supply side poses a severe challenge in that it involves issues and concerns which are peripheral to current practice and so the profession itself may not be best equipped to offer learning opportunities. This is reinforced by the fact that much of that peripheral activity lies at or across disciplinary boundaries and involves other professions and other agencies as was discussed in Chapters 7 and 8. Continuing education needs to become as inter-professional as future practice and future practice needs to reflect that model. As important as these developments is the need for continuing education to be planned and programmed, for the profession as a whole, and for individuals at salient points in their careers. These issues are considered below.

CAREER TRANSITIONS IN COMMUNITY-BASED PRACTICE

In his discussion about professional education Houle stresses the importance of the transitions which occur in a professional career and the need to create opportunities for individuals to prepare for those transitions (Houle 1980). This need is evident for example in the transition from being simply a practising partner to taking on a directive or managerial responsibility within practice, or in the adoption of particular roles within the practice in relation to audit or specialised areas of care. Many of these are predictable transitions, and most could be organised to allow for preparation to be made in anticipation of the transition, though this does not seem to occur very often.

It is ironic that medical education for general practice in Britain is one area where the need has been recognised and to some degree institutionalised. This case again affords an instructive example. The profession has established an elaborate structure for the vocational training of new entrants and has recognised the need for those involved as trainers to prepare for their educational role before formally taking responsibility for a trainee. The educational process as we saw earlier rests on a one-to-one relationship between trainee and trainer and potential trainers are required to undertake specific training for their role. They are also required to go through a formal selection process and to submit themselves, and their practices, for periodic review to check whether they continue to satisfy the requirements and standards for training. This follows an earlier period where this was not required and it was discovered that 'good doctors' did not automatically make good trainers, a message about the transferability of skills from practice into education which has implications for other areas as well (Horder and Swift 1979). It is of direct interest, for example, in relation to health education for patients and the public which is often seen as a natural part of the doctor's skills and a corollary of good consulting skills. It is interesting to ponder what the effect would be of extending the professional education model to other areas which involve teaching and learning such as this with patients and by analogy with other staff in the health care team. It is also worthy of note that the requirements for pre-training do not extend to GP Tutors taking on the much more demanding task of stimulating and developing continuing education for their varied colleagues.

If this model is accepted then it becomes immediately obvious that there are many other transitions which may be identified within community-based care where preparation should be as relevant as in the case of education (Boaden 1997). These include the many roles within developing community-based practice which fall outside conventional clinical activity. For example, there will be a need in the future for someone to take on leadership and managerial roles within the enlarged community-based teams which seem likely to develop. There will be a need for someone to take on the supervisory role with staff who may be given increased autonomy, but whose position may not merit totally independent practice. There will be a need for someone to provide training for staff within the team, and to engage with the development of teamwork which is the hallmark of the new style of community-based practice. All of these are transitions which can be predicted in a career within any of the community-based professions and all are roles which do not flow directly from initial professional training and so require some kind of preparation for their effective exercise.

STRUCTURES FOR CONTINUED LEARNING

These thoughts about transitions echo the discussion throughout the text which has emphasised the climate of change in health care and has involved both explicit and implicit understandings about the character of future systems of community-based health care. In the context of continuing education this poses particular problems. The initial argument of the text was that education and practice needed to be brought into much greater congruence than was currently the case, and that this needed particularly to be done in the context of community-based practice. This requires two elements to be fulfilled. One is that practice needs to be organised in ways appropriate to the delivery of future care, but also in ways which will facilitate the kind of education professionals will need for such practice. The other is the need to construct an educational system designed to deliver that education and to meet the demands which will be placed on professional staff by the new system.

To develop and sustain congruence between health care and professional education both need to display a number of characteristics. They must be inter-disciplinary in character and they must bring together the various agencies involved in the community in ways which facilitate practice and education for practice. In addition, they must provide a context in which education and practice may be effectively planned, managed and resourced so that there can be an active correspondence between the transitions of practice and educational provision competent to deal with the preparation involved in making those transitions. There must be an end to educational reform which is responding to changes already introduced in practice. It needs to anticipate and precede them in order to facilitate effective and efficient change.

On the practice side this is a difficult challenge as it involves either a change in the structures delivering established care, or significant changes in the cultures and working relationships which operate within the current structures. Neither of these changes is easy and both will involve considerable effort in education and training for their successful implementation. Both involve greatly enhanced communication across the boundaries which traditionally divide the professions and the sectors of care. They may also involve managerial structures and resource allocations which bridge those divides. New single purpose organisations charged with providing most community-based care services offer one model, but seem unlikely to emerge, at least not ones which involve the full array of possibilities. The alternative is greater cooperation, but this has been called for over many years without great success. As discussed in Chapter 8, this may require new structures to permit resources to be used in novel ways to stimulate new partnerships and working relationships. More probably change of this kind will rely more indirectly on changes of culture and practice rather than structure and organisation.

On the educational side the problem is more difficult. There is an existing structure for the delivery of medical and other related health care education, but as has been discussed, it is weakest in the area of continuing education especially where radical changes are involved. Such changes and the scale of staffing involved suggest the need for a more elaborate system to cater for continuing education. Many of the elements necessary to such a system are already to be found within the educational system, but they are fragmented and their divergent capacities are seldom brought to bear on the issues of community-based health care and its educational and training needs. In fact the problems echo those on the practice side. Disciplinary divides, narrowly circumscribed budgets, research traditions which inhibit cross-examination of institutions and the absence of high quality management within higher education militate against what is required. Some efforts are under way, but often they fail to address the key divide, for example, between medicine and the other professions, because of the established patterns of dominance which are almost always seen as being threatened by such development. If education is to serve the new community-based practice then it must engage the agenda within its own institutions before it can sensibly assist to address the agenda outside. Some of the issues which need to be addressed are considered below.

SUPPORT FOR CONTINUING LEARNING

It is already clear that the future of community-based practice involves development in areas, some of which are far removed from the core learning of early professional education. In such cases, and it may even be also in areas of core learning, there is a need to consider the support for learners which may be necessary in a more fully elaborated system of continuing medical education. Two elements are involved. One is the provision of basic learning opportunities in relation to areas of work which have not been the subject of earlier consideration within initial professional training. The other is the support mechanisms needed for those working in such areas after they have taken up their new tasks much in the way that supervision and support might be offered in the early stages of conventional professional practice.

The first of these involves several elements which have to be combined to make effective provision which acknowledges the constraints under which continuing education will inevitably have to be undertaken. Extension of the range of disciplines relevant to community-based practice means that teachers and facilitators from the new subject areas involved will need to be recruited. They will need to develop their understanding of the health service through research and consultancy which can inform their education and training roles and enable them to carry the respect and confidence of their professional 'students'. There are already examples of centres where these features apply, but they are limited in scope and sometimes provide a model of provision which is expensive and not user-friendly to those needing its services. Much of this provision hinges on health service management reflecting in some measure the dominance of the hospital sector with its much stronger management ethos. Community-based care figures much less strongly in most cases.

There is also a tendency for much provision to be oriented around the institutional norms of higher education with formal qualifications involved and with the structure of provision matching the conventional requirements of such qualifications. Professionals within community-based health care may need something different. Shorter courses, distance learning with periodic attendance, local facilities to provide necessary contact often outwith the formal conduct of courses, and of course access to relevant material organised in a relatively user-friendly fashion. None of these is new, but nor are any of these yet commonplace. In the absence of a well-established system the norms will continue to see use of such facilities as only for the committed minority, or as something for which you wait your turn and need study leave or large amounts of protected time for study. These are unlikely to be forthcoming so that the system has to engage the needs of learners without recourse to those kinds of opportunity.

The need for continuing support when professionals engage in new tasks is again not a new idea, but is still in its infancy and largely restricted to mainstream professional matters. As a consequence where it has begun to develop it has tended to repeat the traditional rather introspective professional model. Mentoring, portfolio learning, and similar developments are usually seen as being undertaken with fellow professionals which may inhibit the breadth of vision and support necessary to an expanding view of how future practice should develop. This may be adequate for the maintenance, and even development, of what have been characterised as core skills, but the challenge for the future will take the substance of such processes outside that traditional realm. Even within the current core role, there may be questions about how these supports are provided. For the moment they seem almost always to be seen as something additional to the conventional working relationships present in current community-based care, and so make a virtue of finding a peer professional outside the normal work setting. There is of course a place for such an outside view, but established attitudes will need to change and professional development be seen as part of the mutual relationships present in the work setting. This is more likely now that the scale of much community-based care provides a pool of varied professionals able to accommodate the range of issues likely to arise within the mentor role. Such changes in the relationships between professional partners, or among the members of an expanded primary care team challenge much of the current orthodoxy and raise questions about the organisational culture needed in the future.

LEARNING ORGANISATIONS

There is no doubt that continuing education for future practice will have to engage adequate experiential opportunity for learners even when the disciplinary base of their practice has been reasonably established. This principle of learning is well established in medical education and is highly salient to the nature of the new roles which will fall to professionals as well as to the old. This places an added requirement on the varied organisations involved in, and associated with, health care not only to deliver innovative services but to create an environment in which continuing learning takes place.

Future practice, in anticipating and adjusting to the many changes in the context and delivery of care, will need practitioners who can cope with change but also organisations which can do so as well. It will need many more of both who can initiate change and innovate the working practices and novel treatments and preventive strategies made possible by new health care arrangements. For the individual professional it is expected that the acquisition of appropriate learning skills will assist this transition. The same principles must also apply to organisations. The idea of the learning organisation is now well established though the practice is much more limited. These are not just organisations where individuals are encouraged to learn and to change, but organisations which themselves change and develop in light of their collective experience.

Learning organisations have been characterised as ones which continually expand their capacity to create their future (Senge 1993). They are organisations which move beyond 'adaptive learning' which is what is asked of many community-based health organisations now, to engage with 'generative learning' which will enable them to deliver the future. In the more traditional sense they might have been characterised as innovative organisations, but their creative character runs much deeper than would be the case in such organisations. It is no longer enough to free up some creative talents within the organisation to deal with research and development or creative marketing. In the learning organisation creative, forward thinking is not restricted to particular parts of the organisation, but results from the way in which the different parts of the organisation relate to one another and are thus enabled to contribute to the future. Indeed, it only becomes a learning organisation when the contribution of everyone in the organisation is effectively recognised and integrated into corporate decisions.

This is an important consideration as it mirrors at the organisational level those characteristics which are widely accepted in parts of medical education about the capacity and potential we might expect of individual learners. If such features are developed, and current curriculum reform is successful, then such learners will need organisational settings which provide the continuing conditions conducive to their learning. They will accept and provide leadership, and they will provide management and accept being managed, because such factors will be understood properly in relation to the requirements of effective organisational functioning. They will not accept them where they are not appropriate and serve to stifle the individual and deny his or her contribution to those corporate goals.

ACCREDITATION

It was argued earlier that community-based practice had traditionally experienced a low position in the established pecking order of professional medicine and that this in part accounts for the degree of change now being required. If that low esteem is not to be transferred to the developing community-based practice, and more particularly to the extended concept of that practice, then care needs to be taken to establish its credibility.

Accreditation of those who practise in the community is important in establishing such credibility but several traps need to be avoided in establishing a system to accredit practitioners. Effort must be made to establish standards of performance which can be measured and which reflect the outcome of activity rather than the activity itself. Care needs to be taken to include the new disciplines and their contribution in any system which is established. Their criteria will be different and evaluation of those criteria will be different, but it must be undertaken if they are not to be second-class aspects of community-based practice. Minimum standards have to be guaranteed, but the process must be designed to encourage the search for better standards and improving practice. Systems need to be established to handle the process of accreditation and, given the volatility of community-based practice, re-accreditation. Peer review must figure in the process but by itself is not a satisfactory guarantee of performance. In the nature of the new practice, non-peer review should become both more accessible and hopefully more acceptable. If it does not, then the system will probably not be performing well in terms of the characteristics discussed earlier.

Other changes in the character of community-based practice should also be helpful. Audit and research should play a more important role in practice, and information about practice will need to be more available to facilitate the sharing between professionals and agencies which will characterise the future. All of these should provide a much richer source of evaluative material which can feed into the accreditation process.

These aspects of accreditation are not new in debates about professional education. Given the emphasis of earlier discussion, they now need to be extended to the organisations involved as well as the professions. It is not merely that the organisation may greatly facilitate or constrain professional performance, but that organisations which do not display the characteristics discussed earlier should have their own accredited status questioned. If this does not happen then we will be left with systems of accreditation which emphasise the individual professional too much in a context where collective, inter-professional activity is the essence of good practice.

10

A vision for the future

This text has been concerned with the need to bring the education of health care professionals into closer congruity with developments in systems of health care delivery. The growing difficulty experienced in developed health care systems in meeting their needs for more effective, and more cost-effective, community-based care throws the traditional incongruity between education and much practice into sharp relief. This incongruity, allied with the obvious continuing volatility in health care systems, makes the task of reconciling the two systems especially difficult. On the one hand, it is possible to address educational changes which might go a long way towards meeting the immediate and explicit needs of current practice within community-based health care. As Chapter 3 made clear, many of the available examples of curriculum development have addressed that more limited objective but in so doing have restricted their use of the opportunities available within communities in relation to professional education. On the other hand, there is a more radical opportunity in the established climate of change within professional education which might allow for changes which would move beyond current needs to meet the anticipated challenges of future community-based care. This involves a much more radical appraisal, not only of professional education, but also of the roles to be played by professionals within any future community-based system.

Both approaches form part of what can be described as community-based professional education, but the use they make of the community and the intentions behind their approach to professional education are quite different. This can lead to ambiguities with much educational reform being condemned as too cautious and narrow, while any more radical efforts are condemned as being impractical and idealistic. Such conflict is inherent in an educational system which has failed to adjust over the years to the obvious needs of community-based practitioners, but also in a professional system where educational change can be seen as a threat to the base of professional interests and traditional practice. The result is that the more radical the degree of change within the health care system, the more radical and threatening becomes the agenda of educational change. The battle which results can lead to stalemate and no change, a pattern which seems to have characterised much of the history of efforts at educational reform within professional medicine. The position is complicated by the uncertainty of future patterns of health care which means that future professionals, and the education of professionals, must show greater flexibility so that the dilemma is not revisited within a short space of time. An adaptable educational system to produce adaptable doctors is the requirement for the next century. It may not come at once, but could well grow out of more modest beginnings as a new community-based practice is established and becomes the context for future educational experience.

IMPROVING CURRENT CARE

Taking the more limited objective of bringing community-based practice to a point where it can better serve the needs of a cost-effective and equitable health care system, the opportunities offered by greater community-based education are extensive. In terms of the core clinical skills needed for such practice it is evident that undergraduate exposure to a much wider and richer experience in the community can do nothing but good. Changes in patterns of hospital care are limiting the learning opportunities available there and creating consequent pressure for such development in the community, but the arguments in favour of it are much more positive than that. There is no need to abandon established features of current approaches to medical education, but simply to extend them to embrace community-based opportunities where they may be applied. The community-based clinic, health centre or surgery can provide the setting for appropriate observational and experiential opportunities. The community physician with whom students could work affords a suitable role model in the same way as does the hospital-based consultant. In terms of the basic clinical knowledge and skills, these too can be dealt with within the community setting, although there may be a need for associated experience to be gained within a clinical skills laboratory or some equivalent. This is in any case a feature which is becoming necessary even within the current hospital-based education. None of this involves removal of hospital experience, but rather it accepts the need for both hospital and community experience as having value for doctors preparing for either kind of practice.

This requires only modest changes in current approaches to medical education. Opportunities need to be found for experiential placements for medical students within the community but these need to go beyond some of the more common current models of general practice attachment. Short-term nominal attachments are unlikely to counterbalance the natural emphasis on hospital experience. However, there are already a number of examples of more elaborate development and much has been written about what general practice can offer to undergraduate medical students as part of their general learning about medicine. There is a constant refrain within such writing which argues that this is not about teaching students about general practice, but in any case this sort of experience is not about students learning general practice. Hospital placements in the early years of medical education are not about hospital medicine either, but concerned with history taking and awareness of certain diseases and their treatment. It is only the relative exclusivity of hospital experience within the curriculum which makes it seem as though hospital practice is what is being learned. Hospitals are simply a context within which medicine is learned, medicine which subsequent experience suggests can as well be applied in the community as in hospital. That there are differences between the two there is no doubt, but each should inform the other in the education of a generalist doctor. Development of specialist expertise comes later.

If community-based practice emphasises psycho-social and family matters and takes a different approach to diagnosis, then it provides a proper complement to the learning which is taking place within the hospital. Hospital doctors would benefit greatly from more awareness of the community context in which they work and from greater mutual awareness of their own work in relation to that of their community-based colleagues. They would also benefit in many cases from the approach to consultation adopted by their community colleagues, certainly in relation to some specialties such as geriatrics or psychiatry.

Community-based education also offers clearer opportunities than do hospitals to move current practice towards the goal of multi-professional or inter-professional development which is becoming more apparent in the more innovative community settings. If they are to gain experience and develop appropriate skills, students need to experience at least some minimum exposure to multi-professional practice which suggests that training must be developed in those situations where that is taking place. Not all general practices provide such opportunity and some take an approach to the practice of team-work which might have the effect of blunting any developing desire among students to engage with multi-disciplinary practice. As has been argued at many points in the text, selection of appropriate learning opportunities which take this into account is very important.

The same is true for multi-agency or inter-agency relationships. However limited they may currently be in the development of shared care, it is important that students are exposed to different health care organisations so that they appreciate the importance of context for the development of their own, and possible multi-disciplinary, work. Awareness of both the costs and benefits of different contexts for both kinds of work may help to develop both the willingness and the capacity for both professional models. Nor is it simply a matter of positive experiences in optimal surroundings. A period attached to a single-handed practice may serve a valuable educational purpose in this regard illustrating both why patients often prefer this setting for their care, but also illustrating the limitations of that setting in relation to many of the proposed developments in community-based care. Even in relation to organisations which are more likely to be developing inter-professional team-work and inter-agency working, comparative experience of different, larger-scale practices is important. The apprentice model has its limitations even in terms of individual practice, but in relation to organisational impacts, comparative judgements are essential to developing professional understanding and capacity.

DEVELOPING FUTURE CARE

At the same time there is another agenda which could be served by community-based education. This involves an extension of the concept of community-based practice towards what might be styled as community-oriented health care though there may be various intermediate stages on the way to that more extreme form of practice. This more radical possibility has been a continuing sub-text throughout the book and it has been implied that if students were exposed to more extended community-based experiences, they would tend to move along the continuum towards those more radical possibilities. If, on the other hand, the intention is radical, then community-based education will need deliberately to seek out more radical opportunities to provide appropriate learning experiences. These may, in turn, promote more radical attitudes among medical students. Such development may serve to bring health care practice and professional education closer together, and do so around models of practice which may better suit the more demanding health care context of the future.

If such more radical community-based experiences are to have effect there is a need for change within the basic curriculum of medical schools. The range of subject matter regarded as relevant has to be extended to give students the knowledge base from which they will be able to learn from the more demanding placements involved in this model. This echoes current discussion within medicine about the advantages of medical students studying the humanities, with a view to them better understanding the patient condition. It extends that idea to include a much wider range of subject matter and to move the focus of concern away from traditional medical practice. At the same time this change of emphasis means that other skills have to be developed. Like clinical skills, but applied in different ways, there is a need for a widening of capacity to communicate effectively, to handle information of varied kinds more sensitively, and to engage with more complex decision-making systems than those related to individual patient care, however complex that in itself may seem.

This range of knowledge and skill is unlikely to be found among the professional staff of existing medical schools. It will involve extending the range of people to whom medical students are exposed for teaching and learning, but this of course is entirely consistent with the inter-disciplinary agenda for both community-based practice and education discussed earlier. This will pose serious challenges to medical schools. The difficulty of adding new areas of more traditional medical subject matter is indicative of the objection which might be taken when long-established subject areas have to give way to those which appear peripheral, if not actually threatening, but which are central to the emerging agenda of change.

THE FUTURE CURRICULUM

These are complex aims and objectives and require complex structures and organisation if they are to be achieved. It is clear from some of the existing examples of curriculum change that intentions are mixed, and sometimes uncertain. The discussion here makes it plain that a difficult task becomes almost impossible if there is no clarity about aim and purpose. Only when both aim and purpose are clear is it possible to obtain the congruity necessary with the other aspects of community-based education.

The matrix of elements outlined in Chapters 4, 5 and 6 provides the basis for planning curriculum reform in relation to specified objectives. Table 10.1 outlines those

Table 10.1 *The elements of a community-based approach to medical education*

Aim and purpose	Setting	Method	Content
Traditional medicine	Conventional community practice	Lectures and experience with established doctors	Bio-medical subjects
Extended community practice	Polyclinic/large health centre	Lecture/ multi-disciplinary/ professional health based	Bio-psycho-social
Community-based practice	As above plus non-health based organisations at locality level	As above plus non-health based experience	Bio-psycho-social with added dimensions
Community-oriented practice	As above but at all levels	As above but to include exposure to managerial and resource decisions	Bio-psycho-social and evaluative disciplines

elements to illustrate the connections which have to be made. It makes clear that only when setting, method and content are congruent will the particular broad general aim be likely to be met, although of course, as we have seen, there are secondary aims which might be satisfied despite some incongruence. The matrix illustrates some of the difficulties which are likely to arise in moving from the current more conventional approach towards community-oriented practice. Even before those are addressed there are obvious difficulties in securing agreement about that objective, and about the detailed character of the spectrum of community-based approaches.

In some senses the latter may be determined by political imperatives which give primacy to resource issues on the supply side and equity issues on the demand side, both of which carry major implications for the character of health care. It is evident from much recent change in health care systems, as was outlined in Chapter 1, that the professional voice in determining those outcomes is likely to be more muted than was the case in the past. This does not render such changes illegitimate, but may lead the profession to resent their imposition and resist their implications when reorganised health care delivery is being implemented.

If this is the case, the profession will need to adjust to the demands of the new system and this will involve imposed changes in professional education, or self-determined change to meet the new challenges. If the profession is to meet that challenge there is a need, on the one hand, to establish some agreement about the nature of the future health care system and about the legitimacy of government expectations of the profession. If that can be done then the outcome should provide a consensus about aims and purposes which should then allow the educational debate about implementing change to be fully engaged.

The elements of that debate fall into a number of categories. First is the need to establish the character of undergraduate education if the models of future professional practice are to reflect a quite different pattern from that which applies at the present time. As we have seen, the current medical degree has a singularity which derives from the heavy emphasis on hospital practice as the principal career pathway. If that career pathway is to change significantly towards community-based practice, then the emphasis will have to change to embrace undergraduate community-based learning, albeit of a traditional kind. Acceptance of that duality, however, raises an alternative possibility. It could be that the aim should be a more general first degree which provides a broad framework for a range of specialties which become the subject of later postgraduate development. That first degree could embrace the elements which have been discussed earlier, reducing the information overload by using new learning strategies and accepting the need for different postgraduate strategies which vary with the specialist intentions of students. This would reflect the practice in a number of other professions where developed intellectual and personal capacities gained in various disciplines are harnessed during postgraduate training for a diverse group of entrants.

This is a challenging proposition for the medical profession, but may be less threatening than the alternative of maintaining the current shape of training and seeking to bring extensive new elements into the traditional framework. It is made somewhat easier by the fact that the system of higher education in most countries has moved from its traditional elitist and highly specialised orientation. Modular courses and systems of credit accumulation and transfer mean that quite different course mixes are more easily available. At the same time most of the elements which have been discussed in earlier chapters already form part of the curriculum in non-medical parts of the university system so that teaching can be arranged with appropriate expertise and a suitable inter-disciplinary student body.

Associated with such changes, and contingent on them in reality, is a change in the recruitment into medical schools. The extension of the subject base of early professional education, or what might now be called pre-professional education, should encourage a widening of recruitment to embrace people with non-science backgrounds, or with a more mixed profile than is currently the case. In addition, medical schools might begin to recruit more mature students, if the overriding requirement for science-based qualifications was relaxed. This would bring into the medical school a much wider range of experience within the student body with much greater potential relevance in relation to the extended curriculum associated with community-based concerns. It would also allow for more considered judgements about selection in relation to the personal qualities being sought among future practitioners.

Such changes within medical education require parallel changes within health care systems to facilitate the learning process. The developing models of community-based practice will be important venues for the experiential aspects of future education. That needs to be understood within any reorganised structures. Training is not a cheap form of service provision and staff who supervise those in training are likely to provide more limited services than those who do not. The failure to recognise this, or at least to resource organisations appropriately to take it into account, has undermined much current education and training, particularly in relation to community-based practice.

This becomes much more complex if the intention is to move further along the continuum to embrace a more elaborate form of community-oriented practice. The necessary extension of learning opportunities involved in such development means that inter-sectoral organisation and resourcing have to be engaged. Budgets have to be used flexibly across boundaries and the mutuality of resultant learning opportunities for several professional groups has to be recognised. Just as medical students need exposure to non-medical placements so too do their social/housing/education counterparts need exposure to medical settings. Recognition of such mutuality might assist the process rather than the present approach which often sees such placements as irrelevant on any but the most limited basis.

Over and above such changes there is a need for the profession to take a more coherent view of the professional career. If the overall objectives are clear then it becomes much more apparent that a range of roles will fall to doctors within the system. Traditional roles may continue, but it seems likely that the skill mix within community-based practice will change the case-mix of the most qualified people involved. That same skill mix may, of course, generate supervisory needs on the part of other professions which would properly fall to the better qualified, changing the traditional role in significant ways. At the same time the development of new tasks relevant to community-oriented practice would mark a further stage in career development. If the career is seen in this way, then the case for educational change becomes much more apparent.

This requires a much more radical re-appraisal of health care than has been undertaken in the past. It implies a weakening of the traditional professional model or perhaps a much clearer vision of the appropriate professional model for the twenty-first century. It will require courage in tackling the many challenges which stand in the way of effective reform but the rewards could be great in terms of a new career for those entering health care, but most importantly many potential gains in the prospects for public health.

Bibliography

Alma-Ata Declaration 1978: *Primary health care: report of the international conference on primary health care*. Alma-Ata: World Health Organisation.

Areskog, N.H. 1988: The need for multiprofessional health education in undergraduate studies. *Medical Education* **22**, 251–2.

Areskog, N.H. 1992: The new medical education at the Faculty of Health Sciences, Linköping University – A challenge for both students and teachers. *Scandinavian Journal of Social Medicine* **20**, 1–4.

Argyris, C. and Schön, D.A. 1974: *Theory in Practice: increasing professional effectiveness*. San Francisco: Jossey-Bass.

Barr, H. 1994: *Perspectives on shared learning*. London: CAIPE.

Barr, H. and Waterton, S. 1996: *Interprofessional education in health and social care in the UK: report of a CAIPE survey*. London: CAIPE.

Barrows, H.S. and Tamblyn, R.M. 1980: *Problem-based learning*. New York: Springer Publications.

Birch, S. and Maynard, A. 1987: Regional distribution of family practitioner services: implications for National Health Service equity and efficiency. *Journal of the Royal College of General Practitioners* **37**, 537–9.

Boaden, N.T. 1997: *Primary care: making connections*. Buckingham: Open University Press.

Boaden, N.T., Goldsmith, M., Hampton, W. and Stringer, P. 1982: *Public participation in local services*. London: Longman.

Boud, D. and Griffin, V. 1987: *Appreciating adults learning: from the learner's perspective*. London: Kogan Page.

Brookfield, S.D. 1986: *Understanding and Facilitating Adult Learning*. Milton Keynes: Open University Press.

Bruner, J.S. 1960: *The process of education*. Cambridge, MA: Harvard University Press.

Bryant, J.H. *et al.* 1993: A developing country's university oriented toward strengthening health systems: challenges and results. *American Journal of Public Health* **83**, 1537–43.

Campos-Outcalt, D., Senf, J., Watkins, A.J. and Bastacky, S. 1995: The effect of medical school curricula, faculty role models, and biomedical research support on choice of generalist physician careers: a review and quality assessment of the literature. *Academic Medicine* **70**, 611–19.

Carpenter, J. 1995: Interprofessional education for medical and nursing students: evaluation of a programme. *Medical Education* **29**, 265–72.

Charney, E. 1994: Medical education in the community: the primary care setting as laboratory and training site. *Pediatric Annals* **23**, 664–8.

Chastonay, P. 1996: The need for more efficacy and relevance in medical education. *Medical Education* **30**, 235–8.

Cohen, J.J. 1995: Academic medicine's tenuous hold on tenure. *Academic Medicine* **70**, 294.

Deutsch, S. 1997: Community based teaching: a guide to developing education programs for medical students and residents in the practitioners' office. *Academic Medicine* **68**(5), 336–9.

Enarsun, C. and Burg, F.D. 1992: An overview of reform initiatives in medical education 1906 through 1992. *Journal of the American Medical Association* **268**, 1141.

Engel, G.L. 1977: The need for a new medical model: a challenge for biomedicine. *Science* **196**, 129–36.

Engel, C. 1994: A functional anatomy of teamwork. In Leathard, A. (ed.) *Going interprofessional – working together for health and welfare.* London: Routledge.

Eraut, M. 1994: *Developing professional knowledge and competence.* London. The Falmer Press.

Ezzat, E. 1995: Role of the community in contemporary health professions education. *Medical Education* **29** (Supplement 1), 44–52.

Fairhurst, K., Stanley, I. and Griffiths, C. 1995: Should medical students learn more about management? *British Journal of General Practice* **45**, 2–3.

Field, J. and Kinmonth, A.L. 1995: Learning medicine in the community. *British Medical Journal* **310**, 343–4.

Foldevi, M. 1996: Undergraduate medical students' reflections on clerkship in general practice: a qualitative study. *Education for General Practice* **7**, 325–31.

Foldevi, M., Sommansson, G. and Trell, E. 1994: Problem-based medical education in general practice: experience from Linköping, Sweden. *British Journal of General Practice* **44**, 473–6.

Foreman, S. 1986: The changing medical care system: some implications for medical education. *Journal of Medical Education* **61**, 11–21.

Fransson, A. 1977: On qualitative differences in learning: IV – effects of intrinsic motivation and extrinsic test anxiety on process and outcome. *British Journal of Educational Psychology* **47**, 244–57.

Freeman, J., Casj, C., Yonke, A., Roe, B. and Foley, R. 1995: A longitudinal primary care program in an urban public medical school: three years of experience. *Academic Medicine* **70** (Suppl 1), S 64 – S 68.

General Medical Council 1993: *Tomorrow's doctors.* London: General Medical Council.

Glick, S.M. 1991: Problem-based learning and community-oriented medical education. *Medical Education* **25**, 542–5.

Gray, J. and Fine, B. 1997: General practitioner teaching in the community: a study of their teaching experience and interest in undergraduate teaching in the future. *British Journal of General Practice* **47**, 623–6.

Greenlick, M.R. 1992: Educating physicians for population-based clinical practice. *Journal of the American Medical Association* **267**, 1645–8.

Greenlick, M.R. 1995: Educating physicians for the twenty-first century. *Academic Medicine* **70**, 179–85.

Grow, G.O. 1991: Teaching learners to be self-directed. *Adult Education Quarterly* **41**, 125–49.

Grumbach, K. 1995: Requiem for traditional medical practice in the United States. *Archive of Family Medicine* **4**, 756–7.

Haas, J. and Shaffir, W. 1982: *Becoming doctors – the adoption of a cloak of competence.* Greenwich, CONN: JAI Press.

Hamad, B. 1991: Community-oriented medical education: what is it? *Medical Education* **25**, 16–22.

Harrison, S. and Hunter, D. 1994: *Rationing health care.* London: Institute of Public Policy Research.

Hart, J.T. 1971: The inverse care law. *The Lancet* **i**, 405–12.

Havelock, P., Hasler, J., Flew, R., McIntyre, D., Schofield, T. and Toby, J. 1995: *Professional education for general practice.* Oxford: Oxford University Press.

Hennessy, D. and Tomlinson, S. 1994: The new NHS: challenges and opportunities for medical and nursing education. *Health Trends* **26**, 7–10.

Herold, A.H, Woodard, L.J., Parmies, R.J., Roetzheim, R.G., Van Durme, D.J. and Micceri, T. 1993: Influence of longitudinal primary care training on medical students' specialty choices. *Academic Medicine* **68**, 4, 281–4.

Hiatt, H. and Goldman, L. 1994: Making medicine more scientific. *Nature* **371**, 100.

Higgs, R. and Jones, R. 1995: The impacts of increased general practice teaching in the undergraduate medical curriculum. *Education for General Practice* **6**, 218–25.

Horder, J.P. and Swift, G. 1979: The history of vocational training for general practice. *Journal of the Royal College of General Practitioners* **29**, 24–32.

Horton, R. 1998: Why graduate medical schools make sense. *The Lancet* **351**, 826–8.

Houle, C.O. 1980: *Continuing learning in the professions.* New York: Jossey-Bass.

Huntington, J. 1995: *Managing the practice: whose business?* Oxford: Radcliffe Medical Press.

Iliffe, S. 1992: All that is solid melts into air – the implications of community based undergraduate medical education. *British Journal of General Practice* **42**, 390–3.

Iliffe, S. and Zwi, A. 1994: Beyond 'clinical'?: four-dimensional medical education. *Journal of the Royal Society of Medicine* **87**, 531–5.

Irvine, D. 1993: General practice in the 1990s: a personal view on future development. *British Journal of General Practice* **43**, 121–8.

Itano, J.K., Williams, J., Deaton, M. and Oishi, N. 1991: Impact of a student interdisciplinary oncology team project. *Journal of Cancer Education* **6**, 219–26.

Jenkins-Clarke, S., Carr-Hill, R., Dixon, P. and Pringle, M. 1997: *Skill mix in primary care: a final report.* York: Centre for Health Economics.

Jones, R. 1986: *Working together – learning together.* Occasional Paper No. 33. London: Royal College of General Practitioners.

Joseph, A. and Abraham, S. 1993: Community oriented Medical Education in Vellore, India. *Academic Medicine* **68**(5), 336–9.

Kark, S.L. and Kark, E. 1983: An alternative strategy in community health care: community-oriented primary health care. *Israeli Journal of Medical Sciences* **19**, 707–13.

Kaufman, A. *et al.* 1989: The New Mexico experiment: educational innovation and institutional change. *Academic Medicine* **64**, 285–94.

Klein, R. 1989: *The Politics of the National Health Service.* 2nd edition, London: Longman.

Knowles, M. 1970: *The modern practice of adult education: from pedagogy to andragogy.* New York: Cambridge Books.

The Lancet 1994: Community-bespoke doctoring. *The Lancet* **343**, 613–14.

Le Grand, J. and Bartlett, W. (eds) 1993: *Quasi-markets and social policy.* Basingstoke: Macmillan.

Lennox, A. and Pederson, S. 1998: Development and evaluation of a community-based, multi-agency course for medical students: descriptive survey. *British Medical Journal* **316**: 596–9.

Lloyd, M.H. and Rosenthal, J.J. 1992: The contribution of general practice to medical education: expectations and fulfillment. *Medical Education* **26**: 488–96.

McManus, I.C., Richards, P. and Winder, B.C. 1998: Clinical experience of UK medical students. *The Lancet* **351**, 802–3.

McCrorie, P., Lefford, F. and Perrin, F. 1993: *Medical undergraduate community-based teaching: a survey for ASME on current and proposed teaching in the community and in general practice in UK universities.* ASME Occasional Publication No. 3.

Medical Education Editorial (1996) Integration of medical education and the health care system. *Medical Education* **30**, 1–2.

Meyer, G.S., Potter, A. and Gary, N. 1997: A national survey to define a new core curriculum to prepare physicians for managed care practice. *Academic Medicine* **72**, 669–76.

Monekosso, G.L. 1993: The teaching of medicine at the University Centre for Health Sciences Yaounde, Cameroon: its concordance with the Edinburgh Declaration on Medical Education. *Medical Education* **27**, 304–20.

Moore, G.T. *et al.* 1994: The influence of the new pathway curriculum on Harvard medical students. *Academic Medicine* **69**, 983–9.

Murray, E., Jinks, V. and Modell, M. 1995: Community-based medical education: feasibility and cost. *Medical Education* **29**, 66–71.

Murray, E., Jolly, B. and Modell, M. 1997: Can students learn clinical method in general practice? A randomised crossover trial based on objective structured clinical examinations. *British Medical Journal* **315**, 920–3.

Newble, D. and Entwistle, N. 1986: Learning styles and approaches: implications for medical education. *Medical Education* **20**, 162–75.

Norman, G. and Schmidt, H. 1992: The psychological basis of problem-based learning: a review of the evidence. *Academic Medicine* **76**, 557–65.

Ovretveit, J. 1993: *Coordinating community care: multidisciplinary teams and care management.* Buckingham: Open University Press.

Parker, J.C. and Rubin, L.J. 1966: *Process as content: curriculum design and the application of knowledge.* Chicago: Rand McNally.

Parsell, G. 1997: Handbooks, learning contracts and senior house officers: a collaborative enterprise. *Postgraduate Medical Journal* **73**, 395–8.

Parsell, G. and Bligh, J. 1996: Contract learning, clinical learning and clinicians. *Postgraduate Medical Journal* **72**, 284–9.

Parsell, G. and Bligh. J. 1998: The interprofessional learning readiness inventory. *Medical Education* in press, 1999.

Parsell, G., Spaulding, R. and Bligh, J. 1998: Shared goals, shared learning. *Medical Education* **32**, 304–11.

Pereira Gray, D. 1994: Community-bespoke doctoring. *The Lancet* **343**, 1228.

Petersdorf, R.G. and Turner, K.S. 1995: Medical education in the 1990s – and beyond: a view from the United States. *Academic Medicine* **70** (suppl), 41–7.

Pill, R.M. and Tapper Jones, L.M. 1993: An unwelcome visitor? The opinions of mothers involved in a community-based undergraduate teaching project. *Medical Education* **27**, 238–44.

Potts, M. 1994: Rural community health agencies as primary care clerkship sites for medical students. *Family Medicine* **26**, 632–7.

Richards, R. and Fulop, T. 1987: *Innovative schools for health personnel*. Geneva: WHO Publications, 102.

Robinson, L.A., Spencer, J.A. and Jones, R.H. 1994: Contribution of academic departments of general practice to undergraduate teaching, and their plans for curriculum development. *British Journal of General Practice* **44**, 489–91.

Rowlands, O. 1997: *Living in Britain: results from the 1995 general household survey*. London: The Stationery Office.

Schreier, R.A. and Danilewitz, D. 1989: A community-based learning experience for medical students. *Medical Education* **23**, 86–90.

Secretary of State for Health 1997: *The new NHS: modern – dependable*. Cm 3807. London: The Stationery Office.

Senge, P. 1993: *The fifth discipline: the art and practice of the learning organization*. London: Century Business.

Shaw, I. 1994: *Evaluating interprofessional training*. Aldershot: Avebury.

Stanley, I. and Al-Shehri, A. 1992: What do medical students seek to learn from general practice? A study of personal learning objectives. *British Journal of General Practitioners* **42**, 512–16.

Starfield, B. 1992: *Primary care: concept, evaluation and policy*. New York: Oxford University Press.

Stocking, B. 1985: *Initiative and inertia: case studies in the NHS*. London: Nuffield Provincial Hospitals Trust.

Summerlin, H.H., Landis, S.E. and Olson, P.R. 1993: A community-oriented primary care experience for medical students and family practice residents. *Family Medicine* **25**, 95–9.

Suwanwela, C. 1993: Long-term outcomes of innovative curricular tracks used in four countries. *Academic Medicine* **68**, 128–32.

Szasz, G. 1969: Interprofessional education in the health sciences. *Millbank Memorial Fund Quarterly* **47**, 449–75.

Taylor I. 1997: *Developing learning in professional practice: partnerships for practice*. Buckinghamshire: Open University Press.

Todd, J.S. 1992: Health care reform and the medical education imperative. *Journal of the American Medical Association* **269**, 1133.

Tope, R. 1996: *Integrated interdisciplinary learning between the health and social care professions*. Aldershot: Avebury.

Tudor Hart, J. 1985: The world turned upside down: proposals for community-based undergraduate medical education. *Journal of the Royal College of General Practitioners* **35**, 63–8.

Tyldesley, B. and Green, S. 1997: Medics need a caring as well as a curing approach. Paper presented at an International Conference on Interprofessional Education, Liverpool. University of Liverpool.

Umland, B. *et al.* 1992: Learning from a rural physician program in China. *Academic Medicine* **67**, 307–8.

Usherwood, T., Joesbury, H. and Hannay, D. 1991: Student-directed problem-based learning in general practice and public health medicine. *Medical Education* **25**, 421–9.

Veloski, J., Barzansky, B., Nash, D.B., Bastacky, S. and Stevens, D.P. 1996: Medical student education in managed care settings. *Journal of the American Medical Association* **276**, 667–71.

Wahlstrom, O., Sanden, I. and Hammar, M. 1997: Multiprofessional education in the medical curriculum. *Medical Education* **31**, 425–9.

Walklin, L. 1990: *Teaching and learning in further and adult education.* London: Thornes.

Wall, A. (ed.) 1996: *Health care systems in liberal democracies.* London: Routledge.

Wasylenki, D., Byrne, N. and McRobb, B. 1997: A pivotal agency model for community-based undergraduate medical education. *Education for Health* **10**, 311–18.

West, M.A. and Poulton, B.C. 1997: A failure of function: team work in primary health care. *Journal of Interprofessional Care* **11**, 205–16.

WHO 1984: *Glossary of terms used in the Health for All Series No 1–8.* Geneva: World Health Organisation.

Williams, B., Nicholl, J. and Brazier, J. 1997: *Accident and Emergency Departments.* Oxford: Radcliffe Medical Press.

World Federation for Medical Education 1988: The Edinburgh Declaration. *Medical Education* **22**, 481–2.

Zwarenstein, M. 1997: Interprofessional education and systematic review: a new initiative in evaluation. Paper presented at an International Conference on Interprofessional Education, Liverpool. University of Liverpool.

Index

Page numbers in *italics* refer to boxed material.

DATE DUE

GAYLORD — PRINTED IN U.S.A